# Heart Failure Recovery

## by Ray Reynolds

## Contents                                            Page

# Contents                                    Page

# Forward

If you are relying solely on the advice of a cardiologist to treat your congestive heart failure without doing your own research it is probable that you will not see much improvement in your condition. While cardiologists are extremely good at treating symptoms with medications, if you want to cure your congestive heart failure you will need to be a little more proactive and find your own solutions. For the last year I've applied the knowledge gained by my own research and have managed to completely cure my own congestive heart failure.

What happened in my case and so many others is that my heart cells that were deprived of oxygen because of my coronary artery blockage had simply gone into hibernation to conserve oxygen. When blood flow was reestablished to them three hours later they revived but were still in a stunted condition trying to absorb enough nutrients to once again become active. The purpose of this book is to explain to you the mechanism of congestive heart failure and the supplementation that is needed to revive your heart cells if indeed they are still alive and in hibernation.

# Introduction

About nine months ago while at my home in Northern Thailand I noticed that a quarter inch diameter white lump had appeared on my forearm. It looked like one half of a Pearl glued to my skin. I went to the local hospital and showed it to their dermatologist who did a biopsy and determined that it was basal cell carcinoma, the least dangerous of all the skin cancers. His solution to the problem was to make an incision all the way around the tumor at a distance of 1 inch so that he would be sure to get all the root system. Obviously this would have left considerable disfigurement. I went on the Internet and started looking for an alternative to surgery.

What I discovered was that thousands of people had successfully eliminated basal cell carcinomas by simply applying an ascorbic acid and water paste directly to the cancer and that within a week it would be dissolved with no scarring whatsoever. I decided to give it a try and after about four days the ascorbic acid had dissolved the quarter inch hemisphere of the carcinoma down to below skin level. I then watched with fascination as the ascorbic acid worked its way laterally just under my skin consuming the cancer cells as it followed the root system that had been established by the growth. On my next visit to the dermatologist I showed him where the carcinoma had been and how well the skin was healing. He just smiled at me and said "Good job!" He knew about that kind of treatment, he knew that it would probably work but he couldn't recommend it to me because it was not an "Approved" procedure within his medical peer group.

About three months later while undergoing surgery I suffered a myocardial infarction involving the coronary arteries that feed the lower apex of both ventricles. This resulted in 2 1/2 hours of CPR followed by a one-week coma. Over the next three months I slowly recovered heart function and was doing quite well until I suddenly went into congestive heart failure. I was admitted to Lee Memorial Hospital in Fort Myers Florida where I spent a week being treated for that condition. I got to where I could not walk more than 20 feet without stopping and gasping for breath. A healthy heart has an ejection fraction of 50% to 70%. Mine was less than 20%.

I began researching two things on the Internet the first of course was any possible cures for my current condition. The other was a painless way to kill myself if recovery was not possible!

I was very fortunate to find a copy of Dr. Stephen Sinatra's book the "Sinatra Solution" on Kindle. In it he explains the simple regime of supplements that he has used for the last 30 years to help his congestive heart failure patients. I had my wife bring the four main supplements to the hospital and began taking them about three days prior to my discharge. When I finally left the hospital and returned home I was not able to walk up the stairs to the second story without stopping halfway up to rest and gasp for breath.

Within one week of continuing to take the supplements I was able to run up the stairs two steps at a time for 10 repetitions. The main reason for this rapid recovery was that our heart cells have the remarkable capability of being able to go into hibernation when deprived of oxygen. This allows them to stay alive for as much as a month on the meager supply of oxygen that leaks past a coronary artery obstruction. After the blockage is removed and those heart cells begin receiving sufficient oxygen they are often incapable of resuming their function until they also have received sufficient nutrition to develop the energy resources to restart and continue their normal operation.

The nutritional supplements that I was taking provided the high plasma concentrations needed to allow those stunted heart cells to revive and resume their normal contractile function. Now all of this begs the question; "Why the hell didn't my cardiologist tell me about those four critical supplements that had made such a miraculous difference?" The answer, of course, is the same; "The use of those supplements was not an acceptable procedure within his peer group of fellow cardiologists." The bottom line of all this is that if I had just gone along with what the professional medical personnel recommended and prescribed I would not be sitting at a computer writing this book! We must all learn to do our own research and educate ourselves to all of the possible solutions and to dispassionately and logically analyze them for any value or truth that they may contain and when we find that truth utilize it to our fullest advantage. I have completely recovered my cardiopulmonary function and am living in the high Sierra of southern Peru where there is 17% less oxygen per breath. Obviously alternative treatments can be very effective.

Modern medicine is seriously bipolar. On the one hand we have the best medical technology available anywhere in the world. If you are involved in an accident and are suffering from severe traumatic injuries our emergency room services will save you if it is at all possible. On the other hand when it comes to treating chronic degenerative diseases such as cancer, obesity, heart failure and diabetes we seem to be a complete failure. The assumption seems to be that these diseases of modern lifestyle are first of all inevitable and secondly next to impossible to cure.

For the last 5000 years of recorded medical history the mainstay of all the healthcare systems from Hippocrates to traditional Ayurveda, Chinese, and Arabic medical practices have been based on nutrition and herbal supplements. Today physicians receive almost no training in the nutritional aspects of immune system support. And when a cancer or heart failure patient asks their oncologist or cardiologist what they can do nutritionally to help their bodies cure their illness they receive an evasive and ambiguous answer which amounts to "There's nothing you can do other than take your prescription medications." I have been unable to find any cancer or cardiology textbook that physicians use in their training that says a word about the role of nutrition in curing health problems.

Until confirmation is provided by large-scale human studies your typical cardiologist will not have heard about any current research or if he does happen to hear about a small study he will simply ignore its results as being irrelevant. The cost of these human trials for a single medication can be anywhere from $500,000 to $1 billion. Obviously if the study needs to be performed on a substance that cannot be patented and therefore no profit can be made from it this study will never be financed. This is the catch 22 of medical research.

On the other side of the coin the food industry does not want the public to become aware of the links between processed foods, cancer and heart disease. These two powerful industries provide much financial incentive to all parties involved including the US Government to not interfere with the status quo. On the other side of the problem are the population in general who are set in their dietary ways and do not want to change even if their lives depend on it. They would just as soon opt for the simple solution of taking a pill.

# My Heart Attack and Coma

**April 12 2014** Rajavej Hospital Chiang Mai, Thailand

I had just completed the fourth of five cosmetic surgery procedures to eliminate the bag of loose skin my face had become after loosing sixty pounds of fat. Rajavej Hospital really has no surgeons on staff, they just rent out office and operating room space to doctors and surgeons as needed so you really need to do your own research. If the best doctor for what you want done happens to work out of there then great! Unless… something goes wrong that they can't handle in their smaller hospital and you need to be transported by ambulance to Sriphat the giant government teaching hospital across town that has a corner on all of the advanced medical technology. That's where I had a stent installed about 7 years ago.

They had just wheeled me unconscious back into my recovery room when a blood clot broke free from its current position and traveled to the small artery that supplies blood to the bottom apex of the ventricles, blocking the supply of blood to that area and causing me to go into cardiac arrest. This would require my transport to Sriphat during rush hour traffic. I had not come out of sedation yet so was blissfully unaware of this.

The floor nurse down the hall however was very much aware of the alarm that was screaming at her to make a decision. The proper course of action was to yell down the hall to one of her nurses to check the old fart in room 427 to see if he had accidentally unhooked himself from his heart monitor or run down there herself and check. The checking part is very important because once she hits the red emergency button an unstoppable process is initiated which will terminate in her being either assigned to room cleaning duties for a month if she was wrong or a commendation if right. Her hand was only 2" from the button when it got very upset with her and she hit it from reflex to shut it up (aw-shit would be the English equivalent of what she said at that point).

Down in the basement an ambulance, its driver and a couple of EMTs were doing what ever it is they do in between disasters kicking their asses when their alarm went off. For a short sprint of four floors they did not even consider using the elevator, they knew the stairs would be faster. By the time they arrived at the 4th floor the nurses and orderlies had me on oxygen and my gurney in the elevator ready to go down to the basement. We were off to the races as it were. I don't know how it is in other countries but here, once started by the EMT, only a physician can terminate CPR. Statistically only 5% of CPR recipients survive longer than thirty minutes. Because of the rush hour traffic my EMT's got over 2.5 hours of quality practice time in prior to being relieved at the other hospital.

Even though I had fresh incisions that were still leaking they injected clot buster drugs during the ambulance ride, which of course caused considerable blood loss. This was made up for by the nurses having provided a box of one-pint containers of the correct flavor so that the ambulance crew could augment their own supply. When we arrived at Sriphat Hospital 2.5 hours later I was taken straight to the Cardiac Catheterization Lab. If I had been conscious I could have looked over my left shoulder and watched a real time X-ray of the catheter snaking its way up through my left femoral artery to my heart.

Dr. Tanawat performs this procedure several times a week so it did not take him long to aspirate the small blood clot and restart my heart. He then sent me still unconscious to the recovery room where my wife, her sister and brother-in-law were waiting. Our brother-in-law went into the room to check on me. What he saw was me thrashing about on a blood soaked bed where I would spend the next week in a coma on glucose feed. I really do hate it when that happens as your abdominal muscles loose all definition, but at least my heart was beating again. Some would consider that to be the best one out of two, I however was still undecided. Our brother-in-laws comment when he got back to the wives was "We've lost him" everyone then started hoping I would have the good grace to die and not be a non-garden variety vegetable and burden on my wife forever. I could not have expressed it more elegantly myself.

I was, however unaware of this as I had my own more pressing problems to deal with deep down inside of what would be a weeklong coma. In my coma I was located on one of many narrow operating room type beds whose edges were touching one another, so I was able to touch the patients on either side of me, thereby determining that they were clothing store dummies. There seemed to be about 15 of them and I was the only living person in the room. For some reason I did not consider this to be at all strange.

It was as though I was being warehoused with the old furniture and store fixtures. In front of me about thirty feet away was a forty foot wide by twelve foot high series of picture windows with some sort of warehousing being done on the other side. A seven-foot tall robot was supervising some more or less human workers as they unloaded and stacked cardboard boxes. Every so often what looked like a modern fiberglass arctic sled about 20' long would move across the top of the picture window. It acted as though it was attached to the forks of a forklift and was loaded with supplies. The large robot was directing the workers to unload it and then the sled would move back out of sight to the right returning a few minutes later with another load of boxes.

There were restraining straps on my feet and wrists, which I was trying to release in order to make my escape from this intergalactic detention center. In real life I am afraid of spiders but in the coma I had a pet tarantula about two feet long that would pass by every so often so that I could scratch his head. Do spiders even have heads? Meanwhile back in the land of reality the doctors and nurses were congratulating themselves for having had the foresight to apply restraints so that I would not fall out of bed from random movement.

I stayed in that state for about a week, watching all manner of street map like displays forming at high speed in great detail and color on the ceilings and walls and trying to escape from my restraints. There were scorpion and spider like insects that defy description running about on the ceilings and walls. For some reason the area on the other side of the picture windows filled with water, which didn't seem to bother the workers who were unloading the boxes. It wasn't long however before one of the windows cracked and a torrent of water started flowing into my room and I realized that I would drown if I did not get free and leave the area.

I eventually released myself from both the imaginary and real restraints. It's hard to keep a good mechanic down when he puts his comatose mind to it! I do not remember making the transition from coma to reality, it just happened and the nurses found me walking around my bed wondering where the hell I was.

It could be that when a person suffers brain damage due to lack of oxygen, the mind goes through a period of data restoration but at a much slower rate than a high-speed computer. There could be a process of checking memories to find copies that are less corrupted and then combining the two to get something roughly resembling the original. I have lost a lot of older useless mind photos and memories. Their associated neurons were probably scavenged to support the repair of more recent and valuable memories that my mind considered more useful such as languages and technical data.

I thought what goes through the mind of someone in a coma might be of interest to someone and decided to preserve as much of the experience as possible before my memories of it faded. An interesting side note is that at one point my wife came into the room and found me standing next to the bed with a long string in my hand. I was holding the upper end and reaching down about six inches with my free hand, pinching the string between my index finger and thumb and pulling the slack up to my other hand. I was watching the lower end of the string so intently that I didn't even notice her entering until she said, "You know, there isn't anything on the end of that string." I was hallucinating that there was a large spider and I was pulling up on his silk strand as he fell towards the floor keeping him suspended in mid air. Thankfully the hallucinations only lasted for a day and may have been caused by the residual effects of one of the medications they had been giving me during my coma.

**April 21 2014** One week after the heart attack

When I got back home from the hospital I weighed 205 lbs. After a week I was back down to 180 lbs. Most of the weight gain was due to water retention from the week of glucose feed. I started exercising and found that I could barely do one standard pushup. Before the heart attack I could easily do 50. It was not because my heart was incapable of supplying oxygen to my muscles, they just did not want to function. It is almost impossible to loose that much strength in one week so I must have been low on ATP (Adenosine Triphosphate) caused by the poor nutrition during the week on glucose.

Over the next couple of weeks I worked myself back up to 30 pushups and was doing about as well on other body weight exercises but never could get back up to my original numbers on any of them. Shortness of breath and lack of energy were also a problem. I knew that I was slightly deficient mentally. It was as though my brain was a quad processor model with one defective CPU. I reasoned that if I could sense the difference then it couldn't be too bad. I have since completely recovered my mental acuity. Either that or I have lost enough additional cognitive ability that I don't notice anymore.

**June 8 2014** Five weeks after the heart attack

I returned to Fort Myers Florida to stay at a friend's guesthouse and visit with him and his family prior to heading down to Arequipa, Peru where I am currently living. I was very much aware of my limitations and breathing the hot humid air caused a lot of distress. when driving I needed to loosen my belt so it would not restrict my breathing. I did however show steady improvement over the next month both physically and mentally.


**July 20 2014** Nine weeks after the heart attack

After a month in Florida lifting weights at the local gym I was feeling great and had recovered my original strength and muscle mass when I developed what I thought was asthma. I had suffered from it about 30 years earlier so I knew what the symptoms were like. When I was lying down there was a wheezing/crackling sound as I exhaled and it felt like my lungs had about 20% less volume. My abdomen was becoming distended and I could not pull it in and breath at the same time.

# My Heart Failure and Recovery

**August 7 2014** Eleven weeks after the heart attack

I could not sleep lying down; it felt like I was going to drown if I did. I was telling my wife about it and she said why don't you go to the hospital. My answer was "OK, let's go!" Her reply to that was "You mean, right now!?" Perhaps she was not used to her suggestions getting such rapid results.

When we arrived at Lee memorial hospital emergency I was quickly diagnosed with congestive heart Failure (CHF) and admitted for treatment. The symptoms I thought were caused by asthma were really caused by my heart not being able to expel blood from the left ventricle with sufficient force and then expand quickly enough to receive the next load of blood returning through the veins. This caused back pressure in the pulmonary veins and fluid would leak through their walls and accumulate in my lungs and abdomen.

The doctors put me on Lasix injections to eliminate the accumulated water and I started producing at least a gallon of urine per day. I was given a sonogram and my calculated ejection Fraction was 20%. Ejection Fractions indicate what percentage of the blood in the heart is ejected into the arterial system when the left ventricle contracts. They are as follows:

70% High normal: as good as it gets.

50% Low normal: still very functional.

40% During exertion you notice abnormal shortness of breathe.

20% A twenty foot walk will cause you to be out of breath.

A couple of days later I was given a nuclear stress test which consists of injecting the patient with a radioactive isotope so that an x-ray will show the volumetric flow of blood, first resting and then under stress, which is provided by a treadmill. I lasted 50 seconds on

17

the treadmill before collapsing. I remember the attending cardiologist saying "Well, now we know something!"

At 20% EF walking 15 feet to the bathroom would cause me to lean on the sink and gasp for air for a minute. I immediately started searching the Internet for a cure and a painless way to commit suicide if I could not find one. I was very fortunate to find the kindle edition of Dr. Stephen Sinatra's "The Sinatra Solution". In it he outlines a very simple regime of four main supplements and some additional auxiliary ones, which he has used for the last 30 years to improve the lives of, and quite often cure his CHF patients. If you are suffering from CHF be sure to download his book from amazon it is well worth the $9.95 price and has enough research documentation to convince anyone of it's accuracy, except perhaps a cardiologist.

## The four main supplements

CoQ10            600mg per day

L-Carnitine      3 grams per day

D-Ribose         15 grams per day

Magnesium        800 mg per day

I divide it into a morning, midday and evening doses. Once your heart returns to normal operation you will only need to take 50% of the above doses for maintenance. I had my wife smuggle the supplements into the hospital and began taking them about three days prior to my discharge.

**The medications prescribed to me by the cardiologist**

| | | |
|---|---|---|
| Aspirin | 80 mg per day | Blood thinner |
| Lipitor | 40 mg per day | Cholesterol reduction |
| Carvedilol | 6 mg per day | Blood pressure control |
| Aldactone | 25 mg per day | Diuretic |
| Coumadin | 4 mg per day | Anti coagulant |

Within a month I stopped taking the Lipitor because of the intense muscle cramps it produced. I have never been able to tolerate it. The others I have had no problems with and they have proven to be very beneficial.

**August 14 2014** Twelve weeks after the heart attack

I was discharged from the hospital to return home. When I arrived and tried to climb the flight of stairs up to the second story I had to stop half way up and catch my breath before continuing. I still wasn't able to lie down comfortably to sleep.

**August 21 2014** Thirteen weeks after the heart attack

I was able to run up the same stairs two steps at a time for 10 repetitions. I could also drive to stores to do my own shopping as well. Within 2 weeks I was able to do the stair routine 20 times and could have continued but my leg muscles gave out on me. So it went, I kept getting stronger and in better condition through exercise and supplementation.

After a couple of weeks of this I was able to function almost normally the same as before the CHF. This was very important to me because on September 6th I had to fly down to Arequipa, Peru, which happens to be at 7,500' above sea level. Because of the lower atmospheric pressure, there is about 17% less oxygen per breath. Since the cabin pressure of an airliner is maintained at 8,000' I reasoned that if I didn't have any problems when flying down to AQP I would be alright living there at least when not exerting myself.

**Sept. 7 2014** Fifteen weeks after the heart attack

I arrived in Arequipa and was able to walk from the airliner to the baggage claim area and then take a taxi to our house. I spent about two weeks chewing coca leaves every night to combat mild altitude sickness. They are legal down here and sold in the markets along with the other herbs and are used for brewing tea.

**Jan 30 2014** Seven months after the heart attack

I have been here in Arequipa for 9 months now and am functioning normally at this altitude (7,500'). I walk one mile to the gym every other day and lift very serious weights for an hour then walk the mile back to my apartment with no problems. I have walked as much as Five miles at a time but after returning to the apartment I need to take an hour nap to recharge. I figure that I am currently at about 50% EF. So yes, it is possible to have a 20% EF and recover from it with exercise and supplementation.

## Introduction to Congestive Heart Failure

The heart can never rest like other muscles do. This requires it to utilize large quantities of Adenosine Triphosphate (ATP) which is what our muscles use for fuel during contraction. D-ribose sugar is a key component of ATP as well as our DNA and RNA. Unfortunately there are no food sources for it and it is very difficult for our bodies to synthesize in sufficient quantities to supply our needs. When we do not have enough to keep our bodies supplied it is easy to use up our reserves, which causes our muscles to loose efficiency. For this reason supplementation is probably a good idea even if you have not yet had any heart problems. It is inexpensive and might protect your heart if you have a coronary event in the future.

As I continued my personal recovery from CHF and learned more about its causes and treatments, I discovered that I was not alone with my affliction. In most developed countries CHF has become a major financial burden on the health care systems. In the United States alone there are six million people who suffer from heart failure and probably double that number who are in the first stages but are not yet symptomatic. CHF seems to be the final destination of a majority of the diseases that affect the heart. Our knowledge of human biology doubles every four years. Because of the medical advances that accompany this knowledge people are living longer and if they do not succumb to cancer they will eventually develop heart problems, which lead to a weakening of their hearts and then CHF.

## The incidence and costs of heart failure

Among individuals 65 or older 340,000 are hospitalized and 54,000 die from CHF each year. These statistics are expected to increase by 25% over the next 15 years because of our ever-increasing ability to ameliorate heart disorders. Although this allows the patient to live it also leaves them with impaired heart function, which induces symptomatic heart failure.

The period from 1994 to 2004 saw a 300% increase in worldwide heart failure cases. Of the patients admitted for acute heart failure the mortality rates are 5% during admission, 10% within the first month and 20% within six months. In the United States the total annual cost of heart failure is close to $50 billion. Chronic hypertension causes 40% of heart failures with heart attacks in second place with 35%. There are currently two classification systems that are used by medical personnel to describe the severity of heart failure in a patient. They are listed below. The oldest and most commonly used is the NYHA.

## New York Heart Association Classification System

**Class 1:** Heart disease with no limitation of physical activity.

**Class 2:** Heart disease resulting in slight limitation of physical activity.

**Class 3:** Heart disease resulting in marked limitation of physical activity.

**Class 4:** Heart disease resulting in inability to perform any physical activity.

## American Heart Association Classification System

**Stage A:** Presence of heart failure risk factors but no disease and no symptoms.

**Stage B:** Heart disease is present but there are no symptoms.

**Stage C:** Structural heart disease and symptoms are present.

**Stage D:** Advanced heart disease requiring aggressive treatment.

# Terminology

Jargon is a type of verbal shorthand used in an area of specialization such as medical care. It allows medical personnel to communicate much more rapidly and precisely than would be possible using more common vocabulary. Quite often three or four words are needed to replace a one-word medical expression. For example a heart attack is referred to as a myocardial infarction which literally means (death of heart muscle due to lack of oxygen). You should try and learn as much of this specialized medical vocabulary as possible so that you are better able to understand medical personnel when they are explaining things to you. You can also pick up a lot of information about your condition by listening to medical personnel when they are discussing it with each other. Quite often it is very difficult to convey the correct meaning in a medical discussion without using this specialized vocabulary.

**ACE:** Angiotensin Converting Enzyme

**ARB:** Angiotensin Receptor Blocker

**EF:** Ejection Fraction

**LVEF:** Left Ventricle Ejection Fraction

**MI:** myocardial Infarction

**RAA System:** Renin Angiotensin Aldosterone System

**After-load:** (Back pressure) Caused by excess residual pressure within the left ventricle after it has completed its contraction.

**Congestive Heart Failure (CHF):** A medical condition characterized by either or both pulmonary and systemic venous congestion and/or inadequate peripheral oxygen delivery, at rest or during stress, caused by cardiac dysfunction.

**CHF with reduced LVEF:** A clinical syndrome characterized by symptoms of Congestive Heart Failure and reduced Left Ventricle Ejection Fraction. Most commonly associated with LV dilation. LV fills with blood easily but cannot eject it with sufficient force.

**Heart failure with preserved LVEF:** The heart ejects the correct percentage of blood each beat but the volume is insufficient. Most commonly associated with a non-dilated LV chamber with thickened ventricle walls. The left ventricle muscle tissue is very thick and strong because of this its chamber is too small.

**Myocardial Remodeling:** Pathologic myocardial hypertrophy or dilation in response to increased myocardial stress. It is generally a relatively slow and progressive disorder. Most commonly caused by high blood pressure.


**Acute:** The abrupt onset of a disease. Acute often connotes an illness that is of short duration, rapidly progressive, and in need of urgent care.

**Angiotensin:** A family of peptides that constrict blood vessels. This narrowing of the diameter of the blood vessels causes blood pressure to rise.

**Arrhythmia:** An abnormal heart rhythm.

**Artery:** A vessel that carries blood high in oxygen content away from the heart to the farthest reaches of the body.

**Ascites:** An accumulation of fluid within the abdomen due to edema.

**Asymptomatic:** Without symptoms.

**Atrial fibrillation:** An abnormal and irregular heart rhythm in which electrical signals are generated chaotically throughout the upper chambers (atria) of the heart.

**Atrium:** An entry chamber. On both sides of the heart, the atrium is the chamber that leads to the ventricle.

**Cardiac output:** Cardiac Output (CO) is the total volume of blood ejected from the ventricle in one minute. Cardiac Output = Stroke Volume X Heart Rate.

**Cardiomyopathy:** Disease of the heart muscle.

**Chronic:** In medicine, lasting a long time.

**Congestion:** An abnormal or excessive accumulation of a body fluid.

**Congestive heart failure:** Inability of the heart to keep up with the demands on it, with failure of the heart to pump blood with normal efficiency.

**Diastole:** The time period when the heart is in a state of relaxation and dilatation.

**Diuretic:** Something that promotes the formation of urine by the kidney.

**Dyspnea:** Difficult or labored breathing; shortness of breath.

**Diastolic:** Pressure when the heart is relaxed.

**Edema:** The swelling of soft tissues as a result of excess fluid accumulation.

**Ejection fraction:** The percentage of blood that is pumped out of a filled ventricle as a result of its contraction. The heart does not eject all the blood in the ventricle. Only about two-thirds of the blood is normally pumped out with each beat, that fraction is referred to as the ejection fraction.

**Fibrillation:** In cardiology an abnormal and erratic twitching of the heart muscle.

**Hypertension:** High blood pressure.

**Hypertrophy:** Enlargement or overgrowth of an organ or part of the body due to the increased size of the constituent cells.

**Idiopathic:** Of unknown cause.

**Inotropic:** Affecting the force with which the heart muscle contracts.

**Ischemia:** Inadequate blood supply to a local area due to blockage of blood vessels.

**Infarction:** The formation of an infarct, an area of tissue death, due to a local lack of oxygen.

**Myocardial infarction:** A heart attack. Abbreviated MI.

**Myocardial Remodeling:** (the precursor of CHF) Pathologic myocardial hypertrophy or dilation in response to increased myocardial stress.

**Pathologic:** Caused by.

**Onset:** In medicine, the first appearance of the signs or symptoms of an illness

**Orthopnea:** The inability to breathe easily except when sitting up straight or standing.

**Pitting edema:** Observable swelling of body tissues due to fluid accumulation. When a finger is pressed into the skin it causes a dimple.

**Preload:** A measure of the pressure on the inside of the left ventricle walls just prior to its contraction.

**Pulmonary edema:** Fluid in the lungs.

**Stenosis:** Narrowing of.

**Symptomatic:** With symptoms.

**Systolic:** The blood pressure when the heart is contracting.

**Stroke volume:** Stroke Volume (SV) is the amount of blood ejected from the heart during a contraction.

**Tachycardia:** A rapid heart rate, usually defined as greater than 100 beats per minute.

**Vasoconstriction:** Narrowing of the blood vessels.

**Vasodilators:** Agents that act as blood vessel dilators.


**Stroke Volume and Cardiac Output**

1. **Stroke Volume (SV)** is the amount of blood ejected from the heart during a contraction.

2. **Cardiac Output (CO)** is the total volume of blood ejected from the ventricle in one minute.

3. **Heart Rate (HR)** is the number of heartbeats per minute.

4. Cardiac Output = Stroke Volume X Heart Rate

# Cardiovascular Circulation

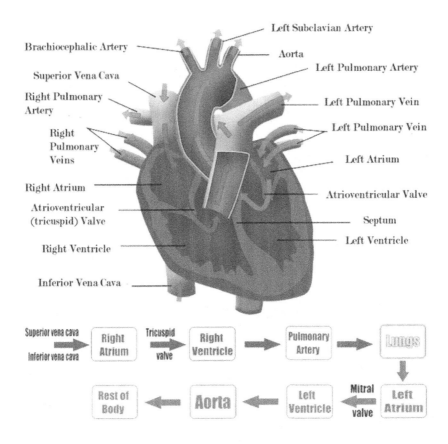

Deoxygenated blood that has picked up its load of carbon dioxide returns from the body to the heart's right atrium by way of the inferior and superior vena cava. The right atrium then contracts and pushes the blood through the tricuspid valve into the right ventricle. When the right ventricle contracts it forces the blood it received from the right atrium through the pulmonary arteries into the right and left lungs where the blood exchanges its load of carbon dioxide for oxygen. The oxygenated blood then returns to the left atrium of the heart by way of the right and left pulmonary veins.

The left atrium then contracts forcing the blood through the left mitral valve into the left ventricle, which in turn contracts and expels the blood through the aortic valve out into the rest of the body again. One important thing to remember is that the right side of the heart only pumps blood to the lungs whereas the left side needs to have enough strength to deliver blood to the entire body. This is why the left ventricle is physically larger than the right.

## The Definition of Heart Failure

"A medical condition characterized by either or both pulmonary and systemic venous congestion and/or inadequate peripheral oxygen delivery, at rest or during stress, caused by cardiac dysfunction."

The term heart failure does not mean that your heart has stopped working and you are going to die, although that is a very real future possibility. It simply means that your heart is failing to keep up with your body's need for oxygen and you will either need to reduce your level of physical activity so that it does not exceed your heart's reduced capacity or increase your heart's ability to pump blood with more force. Personally I prefer the second option.

The seriousness of the CHF is determined by the amount of damage the heart muscle has sustained. It is important to remember that CHF is not a disease in and of itself but the result of other factors that have damaged the heart muscle or valves. Because of this damage the heart becomes a less efficient pump than it was prior to the damage and unable to maintain sufficient blood flow to the body. This deprives the body of the oxygen it needs to support higher levels of exertion.

A heart that is failing usually has a left ventricle that is no longer capable of ejecting its charge of blood into the body's circulatory system with enough force to keep up with the body's current demand for oxygen. The resulting oxygen deficit is what causes the symptoms of congestive heart failure.

When you see a 25-year-old star athlete who has just finished a triathlon event bent over with his hands on his knees gasping for breath, his symptoms are caused by exactly the same problem as congestive heart failure. That is, his heart has failed to keep up with his body's ever increasing need for oxygen due to physical activity. The only difference between that athlete and an eighty year old over weight man with congestive heart failure is the amount of exertion that is required to put him into oxygen debt.

## The Symptoms of Heart Failure

One reason that CHF is sometimes difficult to diagnose is that the early symptoms resemble both pneumonia and asthma to the point that it even confuses physicians.

1. Fluid buildup in the lungs.

2. A wheezing crackling sound especially at the end of exhalation.

3. A swollen abdomen.

4. Difficulty breathing.

5. A feeling of drowning if your torso is not elevated.

6. Chronic fatigue.

7. A persistent dry cough.

8. Problems breathing going up stairs or walking

9. An elevated pulse rate

10. Swollen feet and calves (edema).

11. Cramps in calves.

12. Difficulty carrying groceries into the house.

14. Inability to sleep.

15. A lack of appetite.

16. Friends comment that you are gaining weight.

17. Panic attacks and a fear of trying to sleep.


## The Renin Angiotensin Aldosterone System

When trying to understand the pathology of CHF an important concept to remember is that high arterial pressure is neither necessary nor desirable, only rate of flow maters. The purpose of pressure is to produce flow. One way to increase rate of flow is to increase the diameter of the tube through which the liquid passes. This is why arterial stenosis (narrowing of the arteries) becomes such a problem as we age. It increases the amount of pressure our hearts need to produce to move the same volume of blood an equal distance. Although our circulatory system has pressure sensors (baroreceptors) located in the carotid artery, Aortic arch and left ventricle. They tend to regulate other problems such as hemorrhagic shock. As we will learn in the next section, Lack of flow rate through our kidneys is the main cause of chronic high blood pressure.

Before getting into a description of the RAA System we need to understand what life was like millions of years ago when evolution was designing our physiology. Existential threats in those days came in different forms than we have in our world today. Blood loss and dehydration were the two primary causes of low blood volume. Predator attack was the main threat to life so it was logical for our bodies to develop a way to deal with blood loss.

CHF did not exist in the general population until about 70 years ago. It will, in all probability, take another million years for evolution to get around to adding it to our body's list of things that cause impaired blood flow to the kidneys! Meanwhile back here in modernity our bodies have to try and muddle through with the out of date biological programing they have been given. And it is indeed a biological muddle of epic proportions! The system that worked so well to save our lives a million years ago when we were seriously injured and in danger of bleeding out has been tricked by heart disease and old age into trying to kill us today.

When they sense a decrease of blood flowing through them, which in this case is being caused by a heart that is unable to operate efficiently for whatever reason. The kidneys become most unhappy. They panic and assume that the lack of flow rate is due to blood loss from injury and activate the Renin Angiotensin Aldosterone System (RAAS).

The sequence is as follows:

1. The kidneys release Renin.

2. When the Renin encounters Angiotensinogen it breaks it down into angiotensin I.

3. Which is converted in the lungs by angiotensin converting enzyme into angiotensin II.

4. When the angiotensin II gets back to the kidneys it tells them to slow down their production of urine to conserve water and help increase the amount of liquid in the cardiovascular system thereby increasing blood volume.

5. It also causes the adrenal cortex located on the kidneys to release aldosterone. This causes the retention of sodium and increases the excretion of potassium, which also increases blood volume and causes vasoconstriction.

**RAA System** Na+ = sodium ion, K+ = potassium ion and H+ = hydrogen ion.

**Regulation of aldosterone secretion by the renin–angiotensin–aldosterone (RAA) pathway.**

Aldosterone helps regulate blood volume, blood pressure, and levels of Na⁺, K⁺, and H⁺ in the blood.

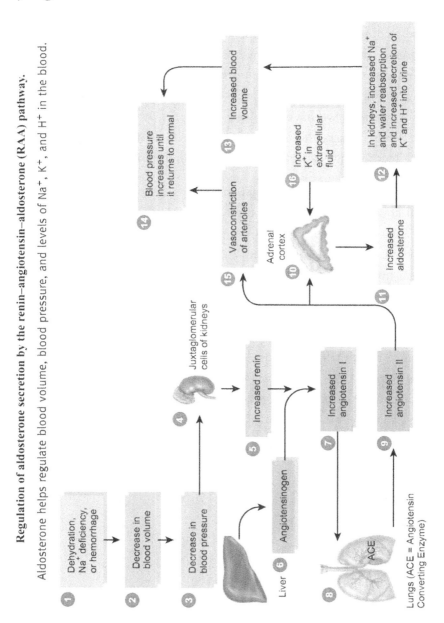

If the reduced blood flow rate is being caused by blood loss then there are no long-term consequences. You will either bleed out and die from the injury in less than an hour or you will survive and your body will replace the lost blood within a few days. At that point your kidneys are once again happy and stop releasing Renin. Your blood pressure drops back down to normal and you get on with your life. If however it is stenosis or a weakened heart that is causing the low flow rate then we have a serious long-term problem, which requires long-term intervention. The alternative is permanent heart, kidney and liver damage caused by the chronic high blood pressure.

All of this creates a worst-case scenario for the weakened heart that could not keep up with the workload before the kidneys decided to interfere. Now the amount of effort needed to force blood through the circulatory system has increased. If your blood pressure is starting to rise, even if it is only 130/85 you need to check in with a good cardiologist. The effects of chronic low range high blood pressure are just as damaging as short-term high blood pressure, probably more so. The longer the increase continues the greater the chance not only of heart damage but also of kidney and liver failure. Many physicians take low-level doses of ACE inhibitors as a preventative measure. Diuretics can trigger the RAA axis as well by lowering the blood volume. This is why ACE inhibitors or Beta Blockers are usually taken with them

## Heart Remodeling

All of this workload increase for the damaged heart as it tries to pump more volume through constricted arteries causes our blood pressure to increase even more. This places demands on the heart, which it is unable to meet over an extended period of time. As the heart fights to provide the necessary oxygen to maintain our bodies it tries to cope as best it can through various physiological compensation mechanisms. These compensatory coping strategies may mask the symptoms of CHF early on but they are ultimately doomed to failure because of their ever-increasing volumetric inefficiencies. In this section we will examine the three main types of remodeling that may occur.

The best way to describe remodeling is that the heart starts out looking like a football and afterwards has the appearance of a basketball. The symptomatic heart failure that a patient exhibits is just the current manifestation of what may have happened as much as ten years ago.

## The major causes include

1. Post Myocardial Infarction remodeling.

2. Coronary artery disease.

3. Hypertension or diabetes.

CHF always starts with an index event, usually a long-standing hypertension or arterial stenosis, which causes back pressure into the left ventricle and a decrease in performance. To compensate the heart muscle tries to adapt by remodeling. This may go on for years until another adverse event sends the heart into its final decline.

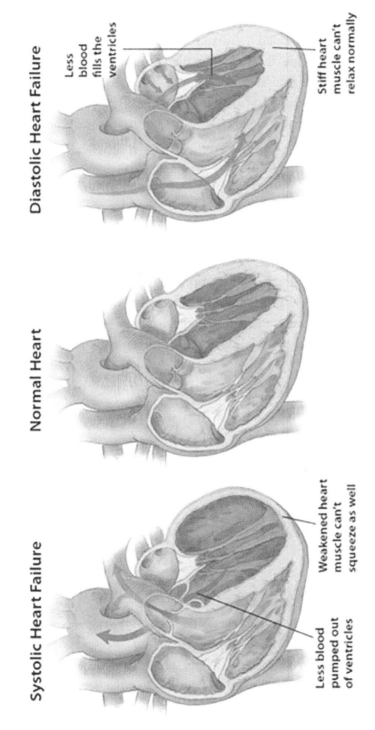

Systolic Heart Failure

Less blood pumped out of ventricles

Weakened heart muscle can't squeeze as well

Normal Heart

Diastolic Heart Failure

Less blood fills the ventricles

Stiff heart muscle can't relax normally

**Systolic Failure**

This is a condition where the left ventricle does not contract with sufficient force to produce enough blood flow to the body. This is usually due to a left ventricle whose muscle walls have become stretched due to excessive preload. 66% of these cases are the result of heart muscle damage due to ischemia (loss of blood flow) the remaining 34% are caused by other types of heart damage such as diseased valves, Cardiomyopathy (diseases of the heart) or myocarditis (Viral inflammation of the heart muscle).

**Below is a cross section of a heart with a stretched left ventricle wall caused by Systolic Failure.**

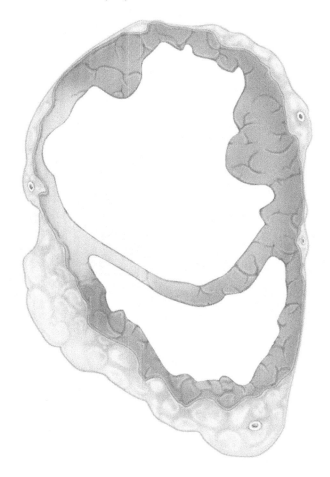

### Diastolic Failure

When the internal pressure in the left ventricle increases, your heart tries to compensate by increasing the thickness of the left ventricle's muscle walls to make them stronger. Unfortunately the heart chamber thickens from the outside inward causing the left ventricle chamber to decrease in size and volumetric efficiency. Another term used to describe this condition is: "Heart failure with preserved ejection fraction" in other words the heart may eject the correct percentage of blood with each contraction but its' quantity is still less than needed to keep up with the body's demand.

**Below is a cross section of a heart with a thickened left ventricle wall caused by Diastolic Failure.**

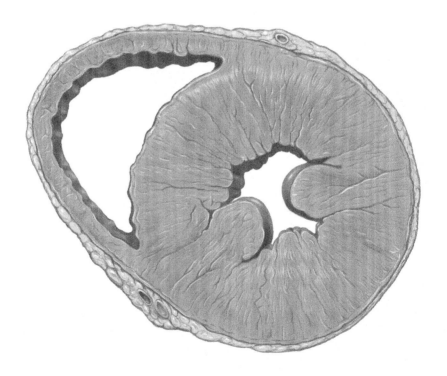

# Right side heart failure

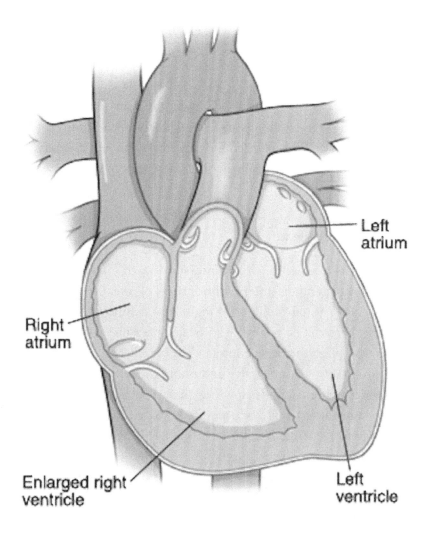

There is a third type of heart failure, which occurs in the right side. This condition is usually brought on by left ventricle failure because the blood leaving the left ventricle is not being ejected into the rest of the body with sufficient force to keep backpressure from building up in the right side. This can cause blood to back up into the right side of the heart causing sufficient back pressure in the pulmonary veins that liquid is forced through their walls and partially fills the lungs causing respiratory distress. Since the muscle walls of the right ventricle are much weaker then those of the left this backpressure can cause either Systolic or Diastolic remodeling of the right ventricle as well.

This backup of venous blood causes the veins of the body and particularly those in the lungs to dilate and then leak fluids into the surrounding tissue. This is often indicated by a distended jugular vein on the side of the neck. Usually hepatic congestion is also present.


## Preload and After-load

Preload is a measure of the pressure on the inside of the left ventricle walls at end diastole just prior to its contraction. In a healthy cardiovascular system with no high blood pressure or arterial restriction there will be relatively little back pressure against the aortic valve so that when the heart contracts a relatively low pressure will be required to open the aortic valve and pump the left ventricle's load of blood out into the body. If however there is a relatively high blood pressure the heart will be required to contract much more strenuously to force the blood out of the left ventricle. If the muscle tissue of the left ventricle is relatively healthy and strong this can result in the heart increasing the thickness of the muscle walls around the ventricle so that the heart muscle is strong enough to overcome this excess pressure. This can eventually lead to diastolic failure as the left ventricle muscle walls become too thick to contract properly and the volume within the left ventricle lessons because it's muscle walls have thickened in an inward direction.

If however the muscle walls of the left ventricle are not sufficiently robust to withstand the extra pressure systolic failure may occur. Sufficient stretch is necessary for efficient operation of the heart under normal conditions. Over stretching however can be problematic as it causes the heart muscle to thin and weaken sufficiently that it cannot eject enough blood during its contraction phase to satisfy the body's demands no mater how much blood flowed into its left ventricle when it was relaxed. Eventually the chambers of the heart will stretch enough due to over pressurization that the walls will become thinner and the electrical pathways in the right atrium will become sufficiently attenuated that the signal our sympathetic nervous system sends to the heart to initiate contraction instead causes a very rapid partial contraction which is referred to as fibrillation. This is responsible for a very high rate of death during a CHF patient's first two years. So while the over stretching of the heart muscle allows the heart chambers to acquire a higher volume of blood prior to contraction it also causes the heart muscle to thin and it will not be able to contract with sufficient force to expel the blood completely. So there is a net loss rather than a gain.

After-load is caused by excess residual pressure within the left ventricle when it has completed its contraction. The excessive residual pressure can be caused by arterial stenosis (narrowing of the arteries) or hypertension (high blood pressure) or both, which make it difficult for the left ventricle to contract. After-load tends to cause heart failure whereas preload tends to be caused by heart failure. It is important to remember that most of our physiology has been optimized over millions of years of adaptation to our environment. As a result the shape and function of our hearts is optimal and any deviation from this norm will be detrimental to the heart's overall function, no mater how logical it may seem.

## Forward and Rearward Effects

There are two different problem vectors associated with failure of either side. There is always a forward and a rearward effect. For example when the left ventricle does not pump blood into the body efficiently the forward result is that the body tissues become starved for oxygen. The rearward effect is that the right chambers of the heart become congested by the back pressure from the left ventricle and the lungs start filling with liquid. Note that the forward effects of both left and right side failure cause the same symptoms. The rearward effects are different.

## The forward effects of left side failure cause the following symptoms:

1. Poor oxygenation of the body's tissues causing fatigue.

2. The heart increases its pulse rate to try and compensate for the low level of oxygen.

3. A weak pulse.

4. Lessened mental abilities.

5. Skin that is cold to the touch.

6. Decreased urine output.

7. Renal failure is a real possibility.

8. Unwanted activation of the RAA System

## The rearward effects of left side failure cause the following symptoms:

1. Dyspnea (shortness of breath).

2. A non-productive dry cough.

3. A crackling sound when exhaling, similar to asthma.

4. Cyanosis (poor oxygenation of the blood).

5. Pulmonary hypertension.

6. Respiratory failure.

7. Right side hypertrophy.

**The forward effects of right side failure cause the following symptoms:**

1. Poor oxygenation of the body's tissues causing fatigue.

2. The heart increases its pulse rate to try and compensate for the low level of oxygen.

3. A weak pulse.

4. Lessened mental abilities.

5. Skin that is cold to the touch.

6. Decreased urine output.

7. Renal failure is a real possibility.

8. Unwanted activation of the RAA System

**The rearward effects of right side failure cause the following symptoms:**

1. Enlarged liver and spleen.

2. Jugular vein distension.

3. Edema of the lower extremities.

4. Distended abdomen due to liquid accumulation.

5. Lose of appetite due to abdominal pressure.

# Heart Muscle Cell Anatomy and Function

## Skeletal Muscle Fiber

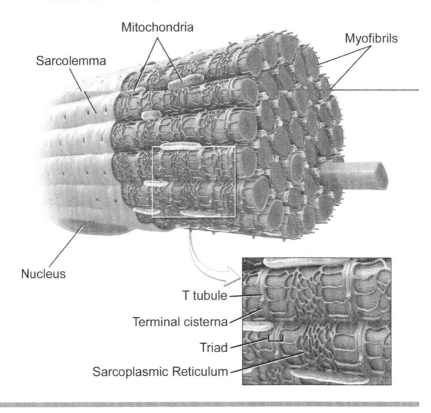

Mitochondria

Myofibrils

Sarcolemma

Nucleus

T tubule

Terminal cisterna

Triad

Sarcoplasmic Reticulum

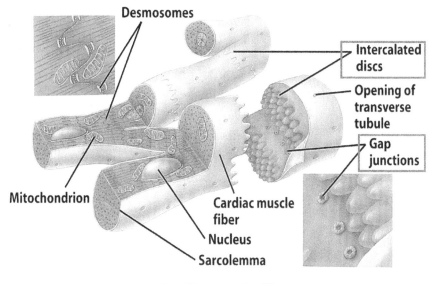

Desmosomes

Intercalated discs

Opening of transverse tubule

Gap junctions

Mitochondrion

Cardiac muscle fiber

Nucleus

Sarcolemma

## Cardiac muscle fibers

Comparing the two photographs above one of the first things you might notice is that skeletal muscles take the form of long muscle fiber bundles whereas the heart muscle cells continuously branch out from one another forming a lattice-like network. This branching is unique to heart muscle cells. Unlike skeletal muscle cells heart muscle cells have a single nucleus, which is centered within the cell rather than on the outside surface as is the case with skeletal muscle. Heart muscle cells attach to one another like Lego blocks along what is called an intercalated disc.

There are small doughnut shaped openings called gap junctions, which allow the exchange of sodium, calcium and other ions between adjoining cells. This is the way that heart muscle cells communicate with each other electrochemically. This process is used during what is called wave depolarization, which causes our hearts to beat. Located along each intercalated disc are a series of desmosomes whose function is to attach the adjoining cells to each other, they function very much like Staples that hold sheets of paper together and keep the two cells from pulling apart when the heart muscle contracts.

All of this creates a community of cells who communicate and cooperate with one another towards a common goal. While we tend to think of a skeletal muscle cell as one long cell with many nuclei the heart muscle cells are truly a community of cooperative individuals. Throughout all muscle cells whether skeletal or heart there are always a large number of mitochondria. The mitochondria are the organelles that produce energy that the cell consumes. Because of the enormous energy required to keep our hearts beating heart muscle cells always have a very large number of mitochondria.

Another interesting structure that is unique to muscle cells both skeletal and heart are the transverse tubule networks which consist of small openings in the cell wall which connect to a vast network of tubes called the Sarcoplasmic Reticulum that forms a lattice work within the cell and allow for the exchange of ions between the outside and inside of the muscle. The transverse tubules allow magnesium and potassium to enter the sarcoplasmic reticulum from outside of the cell.

Once calcium molecules from the exterior of the cell enter into the sarcoplasmic reticulum they find receptors there that they can plug into. When a sufficient number of calcium ions have plugged themselves into the receptors it triggers a spontaneous release of all of these calcium ions on to the muscle fiber tissue thereby changing the electrical potential causing the muscle cell to contract. The sarcoplasmic reticulum provides a means of transporting these nutrients and minerals to the proteins that compose the contractile elements of the heart muscle cell. The transverse tubules provide the entry point from the outside of the cell to the interior where the nutrients are most needed.

It should be obvious how important calcium levels within the blood plasma are. Normally we think of calcium only in connection with bone maintenance, however there are many biological processes within our bodies that require either calcium itself or its ion as a trigger to initiate a much larger process. Magnesium and calcium work together so if you increase your intake of calcium you also need to increase your magnesium intake otherwise the calcium will use up all of the free magnesium for what it is doing and there won't be any left over for other bodily processes.

The next process that we need to look at is how the contractile fibers within the heart muscle cell perform their duties of contraction and relaxation. There are actually two different types of protein bands that make up the muscle fibers they are actin and myosin and if you were to examine them under a microscope they would appear quite different from one another. This is logical since they are made from two different types of protein, which allows them to climb over each other during contraction.

When viewed under a microscope the myosin looks really dark and the actin is a much lighter color. As a result it gives a striated appearance to the contractile portion of a heart muscle cell and in fact we refer to heart muscle cells as striated. Throughout the cell tissue are hundreds if not thousands of mitochondria continuously producing and supplying energy for the cell to use during its contractile phase. The remainder of the space surrounding the inside of heart muscle tissue is taken up by small capillaries, which bring the needed nutrients and oxygen to the heart muscle cells so that they can function properly.

There are two different types of heart muscle cells. Cardiomyocytes make up the majority of the structural heart muscle cells, which form the structural part of the atriums and ventricles. The second type of heart muscle cell is the pacemaker cell, which is dispersed throughout the heart and is capable of initiating and maintaining the hearts pulse rate without the need for stimulation by the autonomic nervous system. They are able to spontaneously generate and send out electrochemical impulses to the other heart cells so that all of the heart cells contract in unison and at the same pulse rate. When we exercise and our hearts are required to beat faster the autonomic nervous system can signal the pacemaker cells to increase their rate of pulse to keep up with our bodies demand for oxygen.

The actual contraction and relaxation of the heart muscle is caused by an electrochemical process referred to as the depolarization/repolarization cycle. The heart muscle has two conditions, it is either contracted (depolarized) or at rest (polarized). Sodium and calcium ions slowly enter the heart muscle cell until the receptors within the heart muscle cell detect a sufficient quantity of both. The sarcoplasmic reticulum then dumps its load of these ions onto the muscle cell contractile fibers initiating contraction (depolarization). At this point magnesium ions move into the cell causing the heart muscle to relax (repolarization). The repolarization process takes much longer than the depolarization allowing the heart to remain in a relaxed state long enough for it to completely fill with blood prior to the next contraction.

As you can well imagine the concentration of sodium, potassium, calcium and magnesium in the blood plasma that are supplying the heart muscle cells with the electrically charged ions to fuel this process is extremely important. Deficiencies of any of these four nutrients will have a very serious adverse affect on heart function. Do not by the way confuse the sodium that the heart uses with the sodium contained in table salt! You will receive sufficient sodium of the proper type for your heart to function by having a varied diet rich in vegetables and fruits.

Under the best of circumstances healthy heart muscle cells require a very high concentration of the needed nutrients to function properly. Heart muscle cells that have been traumatized by a heart attack or are in a stunted condition or have gone into hibernation are 60% less efficient at absorbing these critical nutrients. This is why such large doses of supplementation are needed for the rehabilitation of the stunted heart cells.

## Myocardial Infarction

Let's take a look at how heart attacks happen and progress through the various stages. By definition a heart attack always involves the restriction of blood flow through the small coronary arteries that supply our hearts with blood. Usually this is caused by the buildup of atherosclerotic plaque. The coronary arteries are quite small so anything that lessens their internal diameter causes a dramatic decrease in blood flow to the heart tissue. One of the laws of fluid dynamics states that when the diameter of a tube is reduced by 50% four times the pressure will be required to move the same volume of fluid through that tube.

Usually what happens is that we exert ourselves either through exercise or hard work to the point that the increase in arterial pressure and flow rate through the coronary arteries causes a very small area of plaque to rupture. Although this usually causes a minor restriction of blood flow through that artery it's true significance is that our bodies perceive it as an injury that needs to be protected while healing. Unfortunately the first thing that happens in this healing process is the formation of a blood clot to seal over and protect the injury. This further reduces the cross-section of the coronary artery involved to the point that we experience chest pain.

What is happening is that the mitochondria in the heart muscle cells involved are not receiving sufficient oxygen to produce enough energy to supply their cells. The cells then signal the brain to increase blood flow to the heart. Since you have probably never experienced a heart attack prior to this your brain is very inexperienced at receiving and interpreting the pain signals emanating from your heart. In its confusion it might inform you that you have an upset stomach and you might feel discomfort just above the stomach area. Others might feel minor pain down their left arm because the same pain nerve node that services the heart also services the left arm. This is called referred pain and is sometimes even felt in the jaw area by heart attack victims.

At this point the brain is thoroughly confused by the strange pain signals that it's never encountered before. It knows there's a serious problem but it takes a while to figure out where the problem exists. By this time the heart muscle cells that have been affected by the lack of oxygen flow have started to function erratically and are in the process of shutting down in order to save themselves from death by conserving as much oxygen as they can.

This compromises the overall function of your heart which causes the brain to panic and release a surge of adrenaline into your bloodstream. This in turn causes your heart to beat much faster to try and make up for the insufficiency of oxygen that it is receiving. A faster pulse rate of course will not provide more blood flow through the restricted coronary artery that is causing the problem in the first place and all the time that you've been clutching your chest and thinking about laying down on the ground that blood clot in your coronary artery has continued to grow in size restricting the blood flow even more as time progresses.

Likewise as all of this progresses the area of the heart that has been affected by the blood stoppage ceases to contract altogether with the result that the remainder of the heart muscle tissue must beat faster and stronger to try to make up for the deficiency. Even in this hibernated condition the heart muscle cells will only be able to survive for 30 minutes if there is 100% blockage of their blood supply. However this is not normally the case usually there is some leakage past the blood clot that is causing the problem, which keeps the heart muscle cells supplied with enough oxygen that they can remain in hibernation for extended periods of time as long as the person is not exerting themselves.

When any cell dies and there is no life force left in it to actively maintain the osmotic balances between the inside and outside of the cell it will begin to break down over a period of about seven days. This breakdown is aided buy the lack of blood supply to carry away toxic waste products that the cells produce. When the heart muscle cells break down like this they dump a protein called troponin into the bloodstream. This is a structural protein that is only found in heart muscle cells and its' presence during blood testing is indicative of a heart attack.

So 30 minutes into our heart attack we are really in trouble our heart is beating much weaker and very rapidly. At this point that build up of fluid in your lungs from the inefficient heart function is causing difficulty breathing. Your brain is probably receiving insufficient blood flow to function properly and for this reason you might experience dizziness and disorientation as well. In a worst-case scenario if your heart muscle cells involved in the infarct are not receiving even the small amount of oxygen needed for hibernation they will probably die within 30 minutes. Unfortunately unlike hair or skin cells they do not regenerate. You have the same number of heart cells that you were born with and will never have any more. As we grow from infant to adult the physical size of the heart muscle cells increases rather than their actual number increasing.

The affected area of the heart is now losing about 500 heart muscle cells per second. Once you lose those heart muscle cells you'll never get them back and your heart will never beat normally again. This is why it's so important at the first indications of a heart attack to chew some aspirin and hold them in your mouth so that they can enter your bloodstream directly through the capillaries under your tongue rather than having to go through your digestive system which takes infinitely longer. When I had my first minor heart attack about 10 years ago. I just didn't put a couple of aspirin in my mouth as is recommended I dumped half a bottle in and chewed them all up. Within 15 minutes when I arrived at the hospital I was back to normal and had no angina pain at all.

There are two main classifications of infarctions the first type is called a Transmural or full thickness Infarct because it involves all of the heart muscle cells from the outside surface to the inside surface of the heart wall. The second type is referred to as a subendocardial or partial thickness infarct because it only involves a small percentage of the heart muscle wall thickness. The second type of course is far less critical than the first because you still have a portion of the heart muscle wall in tact and functional in that area even though perhaps 50% of it will have been lost to the infarction.


## Myocardial healing after an infarction

Now let's take a closer look at the actual healing process once there has been extensive heart muscle cell death to an area of the heart wall. If we assume the worst case, that 100% blockage occurred for longer than 30 minutes and a large number of heart cells have died, the environment becomes very toxic due to waste buildup from all of the dead cell tissue. After about four hours their cell membranes start to leak and their enzymes start breaking down their structural proteins and the dead heart muscle cells begin to unravel. However the relative architecture of these dead cardiomyocytes is preserved for a few days after they die. This process of structural preservation is referred to as coagulated necrosis. You might also get some bleeding into the area surrounding the heart from the damaged capillaries. After about 24 hours some very specialized white blood cells called neutrophils enter the area of the infarction and begin the task of cleaning up the debris field caused by all of the cell necrosis at the same time they will send out a call for help from their fellow neutrophils. Within one to three days the task of cleaning up the dead myocytes from the infarcted area is well underway and within 4 to 7 days the cleanup is nearing completion. At this point the larger more voracious macrophages arrive and continue the cleanup including consuming the dead neutrophils who have worked themselves to death doing the previous few day's cleanup. All that remains are the structural portions of the dead heart muscle cells and sufficient collagen to hold it all together until scar tissue has formed to reinforce the area. This is a critical time because in the case of a transmural infarct the heart muscle wall has been sufficiently weakened that blood leakage from the heart is likely and a full blowout producing a relatively large puncture in the heart wall is a possibility.

After seven to ten days something very interesting begins to happen. Very small capillaries start to grow throughout the damaged area providing oxygen and nutrients for any of these cells in the area that still remain viable as well as the production of scar tissue to reinforce the damaged area. Fibroblasts begin to grow in the damaged area acting as reinforcement by laying down very fine strands of structural type 3 collagen. The capillaries and the collagen form a material called granulation tissue. This is the same sort of repair work that is done to your skin and its underlying tissue when you have a bad scrape, burn or any other surface injury. Unfortunately this scar tissue is non-contractile and it cannot contribute to the function of your heart. If the area involved is relatively minor a person might be able to return to normal functionality but if a sufficient area of the heart muscle wall was involved then there's a very real possibility of congestive heart failure later on as remodeling of the heart takes place to compensate for the weakness. Emotional and mental healing can be a problem for a heart attack victim as depression often sets in and the patient feels that there is no hope for the future. This is especially true in patients who have severe congestive heart failure because their mobility and ability to perform basic tasks is so impaired. And of course stress and inactivity will kill a person the same as a heart attack, it just takes a little longer.

# Myocardial diagnosis

The importance of rapid diagnosis of heart attack as well as its' severity and exact location is extremely important. The longer the heart patient goes undiagnosed and then treated the more heart muscle tissue is destroyed and the worse the prognosis for recovery becomes. So let's examine precisely how a cardiac unit goes about forming a diagnosis of myocardial infarction on a patient who has just arrived at the door of the emergency room. This diagnosis is usually based on three major things. The first is the incident history which is basically just the patient telling the physician why he is in the emergency room and what symptoms precipitated his arrival on the emergency rooms doorstep. At the same time that this patient is being interrogated by the cardiologists technicians are hooking up an EKG to the patient to perform an electrocardiogram as quickly as possible. The EKG is probably the most important diagnostic tool for determining not only whether a heart attack has occurred but also the type and location on the heart structure of the infarction. The third most important thing is blood work probably before the EKG has been completely hooked up a phlebotomist has drawn blood and has on the way to the lab to be tested for the trace proteins which indicate the presence of a heart attack.

Now let's take a closer look at the details of the three processes to see not only how they are performed but what types of information the physicians can gain from them. For the history the physician will ask the patient about the original primary symptoms that occurred and then determine if those symptoms of chest pain for example are still present and if so are they more or less severe and has the patient taken anything to alleviate that pain such as aspirin or nitroglycerin. The emergency room physician gets very worried if symptoms have lasted for longer than 20 minutes in the case of a suspected myocardial infarct. The reason for this is that the possibility of irreversible damage after 20 minutes of symptoms greatly increases. Patients often describe a heart attack as a gigantic weight pressing down on their chest or a clamp clamped around their heart and squeezing it. It is quite common for a heart attack victim to describe his pain as radiating down his arms or up to his jaw rather than being centered in his chest where the heart is. Difficulty in breathing is very common because of blood backing up into the lungs and filling them with liquid.

The physician might also ask about any dizziness or nausea that the patient felt. Both men and women experience dizziness and nausea however those symptoms predominate in women.

The EKG is a machine whose leads are attached to the chest surrounding the heart. The cardiologist can then determine whether the electrical activity of that person's heart follows the normal pattern for a healthy one or if the electrical signals are abnormal. In this way the cardiologist can determine if the person has had a heart attack and if so which part of the heart was involved. In the image below each spike on an EKG represents one complete heartbeat. The P wave is produced by the contraction of the atria. The QRS wave is produced by the contraction of the ventricles and the T wave when they relax.

In case you were wondering the letters were assigned by the original inventors of the machine and have no meaning represented by their sound or position in the alphabet. Since we know what an EKG pulse is supposed to look like when it's healthy it is very simple to determine whether or not a pulse form is irregular. For example if the S - T segment of the pulse is elevated to near the peak of the R pulse it is referred to as a STEMI-infarct, which is an acronym for S T Elevation Myocardial Infarct. This type of pulse is indicative of a full thickness infarct which is much more serious than an NSTEMI (Non-ST Elevation Myocardial Infarct) which is indicated by a slightly lowered position of the ST portion of the pulse, which is the exact opposite of the STEMI. The NSTEMI pulse form is indicative of a partial wall infarct.

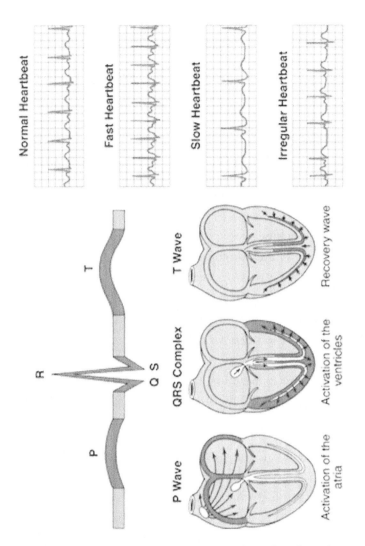

The third test procedure is blood testing for what are referred to as cardiac markers. The major one of these is Troponin which is only found in heart cells. If it is detected in the blood stream it is a sure sign that heart muscle cells have died and ruptured. If any two of these standard three procedures are found to be positive the cardiologist will diagnose a heart attack.

## Mitochondria

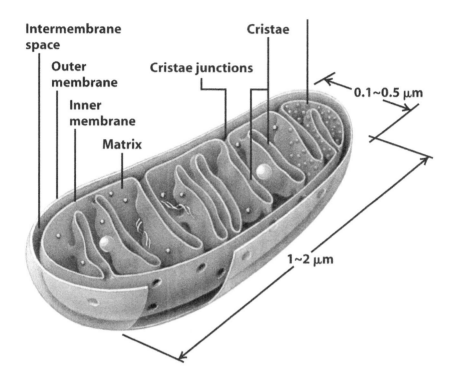

More than 2 billion years ago when life was in its initial stages of development the atmosphere of our planet was quite different from what it is now. There was very little oxygen and the single celled organisms that existed at that time used anaerobic fermentation to produce their energy. Unfortunately for them a new type of single celled organism was developing that could utilize carbon dioxide through primitive photosynthesis to produce its energy much the same as modern plants do. This new process used sunlight and carbon dioxide to produce energy with oxygen as the waste product.

This process was much more efficient than the older fermentation process of producing energy and it gave the cells that utilized it an exponentially greater ability to survive in a very competitive environment. This caused the atmospheric oxygen content to increase, which caused most of the anaerobic organisms to become extinct. At some point one of the very large one-celled organisms, which relied on fermentation for its energy consumed one of the tiny predecessors of our current day mitochondria but failed to digest it. This developed into a symbiotic relationship between the larger organism and the much smaller bacterial mitochondria. The mitochondrion was protected from predators and the larger cell in which it lived was able to utilize the energy produced by the smaller mitochondria living inside of it.

Over the last two billion years the mitochondria have lost their independence from their host cells and much of their DNA has been incorporated into the cells DNA. The DNA, which the mitochondria still have, is almost identical to the DNA of simple bacteria which has a very different shape and structure than our normal cell DNA. The mitochondria we currently have are completely dependent upon their host cell and have devolved from being an independent organism to being cellular organelles that are completely subservient to their host cells and utilized solely for the production of the cell's energy. Without this symbiotic relationship the existence of large and complex organisms such as ourselves would be impossible.

Our mitochondria generate chemical energy in the form of adenosine triphosphate (ATP), which is used to power all of our cells. Cells contain anywhere from two to two thousand mitochondria depending upon their energy needs. Muscle cells normally contain the most because of their high energy consumption. The mechanism by which this energy is produced is called the "electron transport chain", which consists of four protein complexes that work together to provide the necessary ingredients that fuel the fifth and final process, which occurs inside the mitochondria itself.

The first two processes of the four accept negatively charged electrons, which are generated by the digestion of food. These electrons are then transferred to the third process in the chain, which causes hydrogen protons to move across the inner mitochondrial membrane where they are joined by the electrons that were produced in processes one and two. During this fourth process, which occurs inside the mitochondria, hydrogen and oxygen are combined to produce water.

An electrical potential has now been created between the inner and outer sides of the mitochondrial membrane which is used by the fifth process within the mitochondria to create more than 30 ATP molecules which are then used by the cell for its' energy needs. When the muscle uses a molecule of ATP for energy it strips one of the phosphate atoms turning it into ADP. Within seconds the lost phosphate atom is restored turning the ADP back into ATP which is then used to provide more energy.

Because of its bacterial origins mitochondrial DNA is very different from the DNA contained in our cell nuclei. It has a circular shape reminiscent of its bacterial origins and unlike the single strand of DNA contained in a cell's nucleus mitochondria can have many copies of their DNA. Another difference is that we inherit our cellular DNA equally from both of our parents. Our mitochondrial DNA on the other hand is 100% maternal in origin with none of it coming from our fathers.

## Heart Cell Hibernation and Stunted Heart Cells

This chapter will explain why taking the listed supplements is so beneficial for the rehabilitation of damaged heart muscle cells. Our bodies were designed for survival. Many of our important organs are very resilient and are provided in pairs so that if one fails we still have a backup. Eyes, ears and kidneys would be three examples. We only have one heart and it is arguably the most important organ in our bodies. For this reason it has been provided with a very special survival characteristic. Heart muscle cells are able to hibernate if their supply of blood is impaired. They stop contracting and go into a state of suspended animation to the point that specialized testing is necessary to determine if a heart cell is really dead or just conserving energy.

When they are in this state their absorption of nutrients from our blood plasma is 60% less efficient that when they are fully functional. As a result it is imperative that we increase the concentration of these critical nutrients in our blood to as high a level as possible to accelerate the recovery rate of these hibernating heart muscle cells. Case studies have shown that heart cells can revive and become functional once again a month or more after a heart attack. The coronary artery blockage that usually causes a heart attack is seldom 100%. Usually there is some seepage of blood past the blockage, which allows the hibernating heart cells to remain viable for an extended period of time until the blockage is removed. Also there is usually more than one coronary artery servicing a particular area of the heart. As a result blood often manages to flow to the affected area through a coronary artery that is connected to the opposite end of the one that is blocked.

In April 1998 a 57-year-old man was referred to the Texas Heart Institute in Houston for evaluation of left ventricle failure. He had suffered his first Heart attack in 1979. After this initial event he had experienced no limitation from angina pain, and had enjoyed an active lifestyle without anti-angina therapy. However in December 1997 he had noticed increasing fatigue and shortness of breath when exerting himself. These symptoms had worsened over the next five months despite the introduction of diuretics, digoxin and an ACE inhibitor. Physical examination showed a normal resting jugular venous pressure. His apical impulse was faint and displaced leftward. Electrocardiography revealed evidence of a previous heart attack but no indication of a recent one.

Coronary angiography showed that the right coronary artery was occluded near its origin but was filling via collateral flow from the left coronary system. The left anterior descending coronary artery had 75% restricted blood flow at its mid-portion and the furthest portion was totally occluded but was filling through collateral vessels. The circumflex coronary artery contained a noncritical lesion near its origin and the far end portion was 50% occluded. Left ventricle angiography revealed that the lower apex of the ventricles was not contracting and the estimated left ventricle ejection fraction was less than 20%.

Angioplasty and stent implantation were performed, addressing the blood flow restrictions of the coronary arteries. The patient improved gradually over a one-month period after the procedure. At the six month follow-up the patient remained free of symptoms. Repeat coronary angiography revealed no re-occlusion of the treated coronary arteries. Left ventricle angiography revealed improved systolic function of the anterior wall and the apex. The left ventricle ejection fraction was estimated to have increased to 50% and evaluation of left ventricle function using nuclear techniques measured the left ventricle ejection fraction at 53%.

In the presence of even severe coronary artery narrowing, resting myocardial blood flow may approach normal values, because collateral vessels may provide additional flow. However, any increase in heart cell oxygen demand results in a transient episode of heart attack, due to blood flow limitations. These transient episodes may result in impairment of the contractile function that does not recover immediately upon reduction in demand or even upon revascularization. Living heart cells that exhibit contractile dysfunction that persists after restoration of blood flow has been termed stunted myocardium.

Stunted myocardium result from the transient episodes of heart attack, without cell death. The contractile dysfunction persists briefly after restoration of normal flow. Hibernating myocardium, on the other hand result from chronic ischemia and is reversible upon restoration of normal blood flow. More recent data suggests that these two types of reversible contractile dysfunction represent part of a spectrum of the same physiologic process. Studies performed using artificially created, long term coronary artery occlusion in experimental animals have shown physiologic and tissue analysis findings that are similar to those of transient heart attack results reported for hibernating human heart cells in these animals.

Another research trial studied 32 patients with multi-vessel coronary artery disease and evidence of hibernating myocardium. During coronary artery bypass surgery biopsies were taken. Outcomes and tissue findings were compared with the estimated duration of the heart attack. Heart cell deterioration and the likelihood of post revascularization recovery correlated with the duration of ischemia (loss of blood flow). In patients with more than six months of ischemia, biopsy segments contained more severe deterioration of contractile elements, more extensive fibrosis, and evidence of cell death. For these patients, post revascularization improvements in regional systolic function were marginal and global ejection fraction improved from 40% to 46%. Biopsy segments from patients with less than 50 days of ischemia showed less severe tissue deterioration. These patients experienced improved regional function and enjoyed a significant improvement in left ventricle ejection fraction after revascularization of 50% - 60%.

Perhaps the repeatedly stressed heart cell assumes the phenotype of a more primitive, non-contractile cell to limit or prevent further heart attack injury. Taken together, the clinical and tissue studies suggest that hibernating heart cells consist of cells that are slowly deteriorating because of impaired blood flow. The studies also suggest that the deterioration eventually leads to cell death. Furthermore, there appears to be a time window beyond which heart cells cannot recover completely, if at all.

A significant portion of patients who have suffered acute heart muscle damage harbor viable although non-functioning myocardium. After revascularization, 24% to 82% of dysfunctional myocardial segments will recover contractile function. These areas of heart cells may not be detected using routine diagnostic methods.

Numerous revascularization studies involving small populations have consistently reported improvement of symptoms, increases in left ventricle systolic function, and a trend towards reduction in the number of cardiac events. Furthermore, an abundance of non-randomized and randomized trial data established that revascularization provides a survival benefit to populations with multi-vessel coronary artery occlusion and depressed left ventricle systolic function.

A patient with depressed left ventricle function and hibernating heart cells will probably enjoying improved survival expectancy with successful surgery. 33% of patients who survive heart attacks have viable tissue that may not be detected by routine physiological examinations. A variety of methods are available for the evaluation of different facets of myocardial viability. No method has proved superior to another and none is completely reliable. Heart cells that are repeatedly damaged by heart attack will sacrifice contractile capabilities, and will gradually lose contractile function. However they will temporarily maintain the ability to recover.

Restoration of normal coronary blood flow will improve the function of most segments of hibernating heart cells. Symptoms, functional state, cardiac event rate, and survival are improved by revascularization. It is important to realize that heart cell hibernation may represent a time dependent evolution. Therefore, the recognition of viable myocardium in a patient with left ventricle dysfunction and symptoms of left ventricle failure should prompt rapid revascularization.

I shortened and changed the wording of the above article to make it easier to understand. Here is a link to the original research paper.

http://www.ncbi.nlm.nih.gov/pmc/articles/PMC325595/

Tex heart inst J. 1999;26(1):19-27 PMCID:PMC325595

Heart cell hibernation is probably the most important concept to understand when trying to improve your heart condition after congestive heart failure. Because of the inability of stunted and hibernating heart cells to absorb nutrients from our blood plasma we need to make certain that our intake of these necessary nutrients is sufficient to supersaturated our blood plasma to the point where our heart cells have no problem absorbing a sufficient quantity to meet their needs. Taurine for example is absorbed and concentrated into our heart muscle cells at hundreds of times the concentration found in our blood plasma. An insufficiency of B vitamins or magnesium can actually cause congestive heart failure. If you are reading this and do not as yet have heart failure it might be a good idea for you to start taking the various supplements discussed in this book as a means of prevention.

## Diagnostic testing for CHF

**X-Ray:** Used to check for enlargement of the heart and pulmonary edema.

**Echo-cardiography:** Shows real time function of heart. It can also estimate the ejection fraction. The technician can stop the video of the beating heart and trace around the left ventricle with the mouse cursor when it is filled with blood and again when it is contracted. The computer can then determine the volume differential between the two and calculate the approximate ejection fraction.

**BNP Blood Test:** Higher levels of BNP are released with increased stretching of the heart muscle. A BNP less than or equal to 100 is normal whereas a BNP level greater than or equal to 300 is indicative of CHF. BNP helps to increase urine production and regulate both preload and after-load. Complete Blood and Metabolic Panels are also given to check for renal and hepatic function as well as electrolytes and anemia.

**EKG:** To check for arrhythmia

**Nuclear Stress Test:** To determine difference between rested and stressed blood flow.

## Inpatient and Outpatient Treatment of CHF

### Inpatient Treatment

1. Maintenance of blood oxygen saturation greater than 90%.

2. Diuretics usually Lasix are given either by IV injection or IV drip.

3. The intake and output of fluids are closely monitored.

4. Weight monitoring to determine if water is being retained.

5. Cardioverter Defibrillator implantation if needed.

6. Catheter ablation is a low risk procedure used to destroy parts of an abnormal electrical pathway that is causing a heart rhythm problem. During this procedure the doctor inserts a catheter into the groin area up through the artery into the heart. They eliminate the unwanted pathway by placing the catheter along it and applying heat to the area, causing it to be destroyed.

## Treatment after discharge

1. Daily weight monitoring to determine if water retention is increasing.

2. Adherence to a diet regime to promote fat loss.

3. Daily exercise to preserve muscle mass.

4. Medications must be taken as scheduled.

5. The patient should be monitored for signs of depression.

6. Elimination of sodium and excess fluids through use of diuretics

7. Interruption of the RAA system through use of ACE or ARB inhibitors, which produce more vasodilation, which decreases afterload. Less sodium and fluid retention decreases preload.

8. If needed cardio selective Beta-Blockers such as Atenolol and Metoprolol are prescribed.

## CHF Medications

The cardiologist who is treating you probably does not believe that you will live longer than five more years. Therefore he will not be very concerned about the long-term side effects of the medications that he prescribes to you. It can be very difficult to reduce the dosages of Warfarin and Beta Blockers after an extended period of use. If you decide to reduce the amount of these medications you take it might be difficult. This process of reduction is best carried out very slowly over an extended period of time and with the help of a good cardiologist who can check for adverse reactions. The main purpose of all congestive heart failure treatments is the elimination of edema. If you cure the edema you have cured the heart failure. The overall goal of all of these medications is to reduce pulmonary back pressure and by doing so pulmonary edema by:

1. Increasing the force with which the heart is able to contract.

2. Reducing systemic vascular resistance through vasodilation.

3. Increasing the left ventricle ejection fraction.

4. Increasing stroke volume.

## Angiotensin-Converting Enzyme (ACE) inhibitors

Currently the most popular and reliable medication for CHF this category of drugs both reduce the symptoms and need for hospitalization while also prolonging life expectancy. They cause the blood vessels to dilate reducing the load on the heart and also help the kidneys excrete excess water, which reduces the amount of work the heart needs to do. Patients receiving ace inhibitors have a 40% higher survival rate than non-recipients. ACE Inhibitors provide the following benefits.

1. Reduces reabsorption of sodium in the kidneys.

2. Reduces back pressure in pulmonary arteries and as a result reduces pulmonary edema.

3. Reduces the amount of blood in the left ventricle

ACE inhibitors are recommended for routine administration to all symptomatic and asymptomatic patients with LVEF of less than 40%. ACE inhibitors work very well and are the primary treatment for CHF, however in patients who cannot tolerate them due to a persistent cough, ARB's are recommended. If the patient cannot tolerate ARB's a combination of hydralazine and oral nitrate is often substituted. Adverse effects are dry cough, potassium loss and low blood pressure. They are contraindicated in pregnancy.

The oral nitrate and hydralazine should also be considered for patients who have high potassium levels or renal insufficiency when on ACE inhibitors since the same problems are likely to occur when using ARB's.

**ACE Inhibitors with Normal Starting and Target Doses**

| Name | Starting Dose | Target Dose |
| --- | --- | --- |
| Captopril | 6.25 mg 3xday | 50 mg 3xday |
| Enalapril | 2.5 mg  2xday | 10 mg 2xday |
| Fosinopril | 7 mg  per day | 80 mg per day |
| Lisinapril | 3 mg per day | 20 mg per day |
| Quinapril | 5 mg 2xday | 80 mg 2xday |
| Ramipril | 1 mg 2xday | 4 mg 2xday |
| Trandolapril | 1 mg 2xday | 4 mg 2xday |

**Angiotensin II Receptor Blockers**

This variation of the ACE inhibitor is prescribed to patients who cannot tolerate ACE inhibitors because of the dry cough they produce.

ARBs with Normal Starting and Target Doses

| Name | Starting Dose | Target Dose |
| --- | --- | --- |
| Candesartan | 6 mg per day | 32 mg per day |
| Losartan | 12-25 mg per day | 150 mg per day |
| Valsartan | 40 mg 2xday | 160 mg 2xday |

## Beta-blockers

This type of drug is especially beneficial for patients who have had heart attacks that damaged the heart muscle. Quite often they are prescribed in conjunction with ACE inhibitors to treat severe CHF cases.

They reduce heart rate allowing more time for systolic filling which increases both the left ventricle ejection fraction and at the same time increases the stroke volume. It is also a vasodilator, which reduces the back pressure into the left ventricle.

The dose needs to be carefully monitored and adjusted to suit individual patient needs. They actually improve heart function but should only be started after the patient's symptoms have been stabilized using ace inhibitors and intravenous diuretics. Patients with asthma should use metoprolol. The best time to introduce Beta Blockers is during the final period of hospitalization at a low dose just prior to discharge.

The dosage can then be increased gradually at two-week intervals until the correct dosage is determined. Once started Beta Blockers should not be stopped abruptly. If they are discontinued, especially after long time use, they can result in a worsening of the heart's condition unless the dosage is reduced very slowly. A combination of a Beta-Blocker and an ace inhibitor is recommended for asymptomatic patients with LVEF less than 40%.

Beta Blockers with Normal Starting and Target Doses

| Name | Starting Dose | Target Dose |
|---|---|---|
| Bisoprolol | 1.25 mg per day | 10 mg per day |
| Carvedilol | 3.12 mg per day | 25 mg per day |
| Metoprolol | 12 mg per day | 100 mg per day |

## Diuretics

These medications cause the kidneys to become more active, thereby eliminating excess fluid buildup from a patient's body. Injectable Lasix is the most effective and most often used in hospitals to quickly dry patients out. A possible side effect of diuretics is that they tend to move potassium out of a patient's body so that potassium supplementation may be needed. An alternative is to use a potassium sparing diuretic such as spironolactone or triamterene. I produced a gallon of urine in the first 24 hours of my hospital stay and it was another five days before I had lost enough liquid from my abdomen and lungs so that I could actually sleep lying down! There are two basic classes of diuretics.

Loop Diuretics such as Bumetanide, Ethacrynic acid and Furosemide (Lasix) have the effect of reducing heart preload by reducing the amount of blood volume in the left ventricle. This in turn reduces pressure in the pulmonary arteries there by reducing pulmonary edema. They are contraindicated in pregnancy. Potassium sparing diuretics are the ones most often prescribed as they help to maintain the patients potassium levels which aids in lowering blood pressure.

Potassium sparing diuretics with normal starting and target doses

| Trade Name | Starting Dose | Target Dose | Duration |
|---|---|---|---|
| Spironolactone | 12.5 per day | 50 mg per day | 48 hrs |
| Eplerenone | 25 mg per day | 100 mg per day | |
| Amilioride | 5 mg per day | 20 mg per day | 24 hrs |
| Triamterene | 50 mg 2xday | 100 mg 2xday | 8 hrs |

## Vasodilators

**Nitroglycerin:** This type is time released and its effects last for hours.

**Isosorbide:** Is long acting and is used for outpatient treatment.

**Hydralazine:** is also long acting and used for outpatient treatment.

**Nitroprusside:** Only used in emergencies.

## Anticoagulants

These drugs help prevent the formation of clots especially inside the heart chambers. The most commonly prescribed anticoagulants are Heparin, Warfarin and Coumadin. The dosage must be carefully monitored to determine the correct strength. If the dosage is too high bleeding inside the nasal passages and gums may occur.

## Positive inotropic drugs

This type of drug is sometimes used on patients who have severe symptoms and are not responding well to the more common treatments. They cause muscles to contract with more force. This is a "when all else fails option" Some of the most popular ones are; Inamrinone, Dobutamine, Dopamine and Milrinone

## LCZ696

This is the first medication in 20 years that has produced a significant increase in efficacy over the older drugs such as ACE inhibitors. In a recent 27 month double blind clinical trial, with close to 9,000 CHF patients with reduced ejection fractions in 47 countries. The trial showed that LCZ696:

1. Reduced deaths from cardiovascular causes by 20 percent.

2. Reduced heart failure hospitalizations by 21 percent.

3. Reduced the risk of all cause mortality by 16 percent.

What is more remarkable is that the control group received Enalapril the current medication of choice for treating low ejection fractions. So those percentages indicate how much more effective it was over the Enalapril and without serious side effects. The data was so compelling that an ethics council monitoring the trial data requested that the study end seven months early to expedite earlier release to patients. It should be available in the US in 2015. Novartis is the manufacturer. LCZ696 combines two blood pressure drugs an angiotensin II receptor blocker (ARB) and the neprilysin inhibitor known as sacubitril. Here's a link to a pdf of the research paper.

http://www.nejm.org/doi/pdf/10.1056/NEJMoa1409077

## Stem cell research

The most promising area of heart failure research is in the development of stem cell therapies designed to repair the heart muscle at a cellular level. In January 17, 2011 Mesoblast completed successful phase 2 trials of their proprietary stem cell treatment Revascor for congestive heart failure. This placebo-controlled trial involved 60 heart failure patients who received Revascor as a single injection at one of three dosage strengths plus standard of care. The control group received standard of care alone. After six months the following results were reported:

Less than one half of the patients who received Revascor developed adverse cardiac events over the follow-up period.

Revascor also reduced the number of patients who developed any major cardiac events from 40% to 6.7%

A single injection of Revascor reduced the overall monthly rate of major coronary events by 84% compared with the control group.

Every dosage tested demonstrated the same protective effect.

The overall monthly rate of cardiac-related hospitalizations was reduced by 48%

There have been no adverse side effects at any of the doses tested. Last year Revascor entered phase 3 trials, which should conclude in 2015.

## Implantable Cardioverter Defibrillator

This device is often implanted under the skin on the left side of the upper chest. It is two inches square and has a pair of wires that enter the heart through an artery and are attached to the inner surface of the right atrium. A battery that is good for about 10 years powers it. If your heart goes into fibrillation the ICD applies an electrical shock to restore normal heart rhythm.

## Pericardial Restraint Devices

These are mesh sleeves that are inserted through a small incision in the left abdominal area and placed over the exterior of dilated hearts to keep them from ballooning excessively.

## Ventricular Assist Devices

These are small pumps, which are plumbed into the left ventricle to assist it in pumping blood throughout the body. They are powered by a battery pack that is located outside of the abdominal cavity.

## MED (Minimum Effective Dose)

This is a very fundamental and necessary concept to understand. Cardiologists and other physicians have been programed to prescribe prescription medications in as large a quantity as possible. If a little is good then more must be better. However as individuals we all vary in our tolerance of medications as well as our response to them. If you get up in the morning, measure your blood pressure/pulse rate and they are 105/75 X 65 the question becomes why would you need to take medications designed to reduce your blood pressure and pulse rate?

What I normally do under those circumstances is continue on with my day and test my blood pressure every couple of hours. When it starts to go up I take the medications to keep it from rising any further. If I have a very active day and am getting sufficient exercise I may not need to take the morning dose at all but can wait until 6 PM and take my evening dose. Every day is different so be sure to tailor your intake of any prescription medications to your symptoms and not to some arbitrary schedule that a physician has given you.

Also as you loose fat and the supplementation starts to have its' effect you may find that your numbers are too low and you will need to reduce the amount of the prescription medications you are taking to compensate. Fish oil and vitamin E are powerful blood thinners that can be used to lower your dependence on prescription thinners. If you are worried about aspirin causing stomach problems chew it up and hold it in your mouth for about 10 minutes and it will be absorbed directly into your blood.

# Signs of Magnesium Deficiency

Magnesium is an essential mineral our bodies cannot manufacture so it must be obtained through diet. Most people in the United States have a magnesium deficiency which interferes with nearly 20,000 biological processes within their bodies. What I'm going to do in this chapter is present some diagnostic tools that you can use to determine if your obtaining sufficient magnesium, calcium and potassium in your diet. Your heart muscle cells contract and relax according to their electrical charge either positive or negative.

In order to create these alternating charges your heart muscle cells must take in and expel magnesium and calcium ions at the same rate that the hearts beats. This requires an incredibly large quantity of these minerals in our blood plasma in order to create the 100,000 pulses per day that our hearts must generate to keep us alive let alone all of the other critical processes that magnesium facilitates throughout our bodies.

Chronic low level stress is one of the main contributors to magnesium deficiency. Whether it is caused by interpersonal relationships, job problems or just the general stress of living in a large city in these modern times, stress is not simply an emotional condition. It also promotes physiological changes within our bodies one of which is the secretion of cortisol. When it becomes impossible for us to resolve the issues which are causing our stress we then have a constant and steady drip of cortisol entering our bloodstream.

This interferes with the proper function of our bodies by shutting down our immune systems along with countless other biological processes that it considers unnecessary so that we can use that energy for the fight or flight response to danger. 15,000 years ago the stress was over in less than 30 minutes and you were either dead or out of danger. If only it was that simple today.

Another little known cause of magnesium deficiency is diuretics.

Drinking several cups of caffeinated coffee each day produces a major loss of magnesium. However on the plus side it also decreases your chance of having cancer by 40% so don't necessarily stop drinking coffee to conserve magnesium just supplement enough magnesium to make up for your magnesium losses and keep the coffee. Obviously if you have congestive heart failure drinking a beverage which causes your blood vessels to constrict might not be a good idea in the first place!

One possible scenario would be to drink your coffee in the morning then wait a couple of hours until it's out of your system, then take your magnesium supplement and obtain the benefits of it for the remainder of the day. In most of the developed world especially the United States the main contributor to magnesium deficiency is our diets. Mainly because of the high consumption of refined carbohydrates especially sugar.

One of the most prevalent symptoms of magnesium deficiency is depression, which judging by the record sales of antidepressants in the US seems to be at epidemic levels. Another symptom of magnesium deficiency is high blood pressure. Magnesium causes our blood vessels to dilate thereby reducing blood pressure. An insufficiency of magnesium has the opposite effect so if you have high blood pressure one of the first things you do is supplement magnesium and see if that corrects the problem. Another manifestation of low magnesium levels are migraine headaches. In a large percentage of cases supplementation of magnesium eliminates or greatly reduces the frequency of migraines.

If a person has high blood pressure due to low levels of magnesium his cardiologist will assume that it is being caused by his RAA System and will prescribe a diuretic to reduce the quantity of blood that his heart has to pump. The diuretic then reduces the patient's magnesium level even further and produces the opposite of the effect that was intended. Almost everyone knows to supplement calcium as a preventative for bone loss. What they do not realize is that magnesium and calcium are synergistic and must be used together by our bodies to enable many of the benefits that we attribute solely to calcium supplementation. The magnesium is a critical component in the mineralization of the outer hard layers of our bones so you can take all the calcium you want but if you are not at the same time consuming enough magnesium you will still have osteoporosis.

Another indication of low magnesium levels is muscle twitching or spasms. If you have an overly high blood viscosity this can also be caused by low magnesium levels. The easiest way to deal with high blood viscosity levels is to simply donate a pint of blood every three months which will probably be just as effective at thinning your blood as the prescription medications such as warfarin but will be far less detrimental to your health.


**Natural Ways to Lower Your blood Pressure**

In the short term high blood pressure medications are both very effective and necessary because the first thing you want to do is get that blood pressure down to an acceptable level as fast as you can. However in the long run there are alternative natural treatments, which are more affective and safer. The first thing that a person with high blood pressure needs to do is to go through the list of probable causes and determine if any of them apply to him. Usually you will find two or three that are possible causes for your hypertension. The next step is to try and eliminate these causes from your life.

The first thing you need to know is that studies have shown conclusively that the prevalence of hypertension increases proportionately to the distance a particular population is from the equator. In other words people who live close to the equator regardless of their race or ethnicity have a much lower occurrence per capita of hypertension than populations who live in more temperate northern and southern portions of the hemispheres. This is probably caused by a decrease in solar radiation striking the skin and causing the creation of vitamin D. Usually there is more cloud cover north and south of the equator especially during the wintertime. Also because it is colder for six months out of the year the majority of the population wears heavy clothing that does not allow the solar radiation to contact their skin and produce the needed vitamin D.

Research studies by the pharmaceutical companies themselves have indicated that vitamin D is just as effective as ACE inhibitors at reducing blood pressure and the only reason they do not recommend the use of vitamin D instead is that they cannot patent vitamin D as it is a naturally occurring vitamin. So their work around was to develop a patentable chemical that would perform the same function as vitamin D does but at a different location within our bodies. In this same research study the pharmaceutical research scientist concluded that what they really needed to do was come up with an analog for vitamin D that was sufficiently different from the natural version that they could patent it and use it instead because it was more effective than the ace inhibitors. This process of supplementation with vitamin D3 usually takes three months before your blood pressure starts coming down and another three months before it's down to where it should be.

The next problem that might be causing your hypertension is heavy metal contamination. Everyone in the world including the Penguins in Antarctica have heavy metal contamination. Because of manufacturing and poor regulation heavy metal contamination has become a worldwide problem even in pristine locations where no manufacturing exists. One of the problems with detecting heavy metal contamination in a person's body is that the majority of it is located in the bones rather than the bloodstream so that a simple blood test will not give you a proper indication of reality. The only way you can effectively determine the quantity of heavy metals your body contains is to undergo a one time chelation therapy to draw those heavy metals out of their resting place in your bones into your bloodstream where the kidneys can remove them and then your urine can be tested to determine your actual level of contamination. You will probably find that you will need to undergo a complete series of chelation in order to remove the lead, arsenic, cadmium, mercury and other types of heavy metals. Chelation therapy has also been proven to reduce the death rate in diabetics by 40%.

High levels of blood insulin will also cause high blood pressure as well as stimulating the liver to produce more cholesterol than is needed. So if you're a type II diabetic who has out-of-control insulin production then that would be the next problem to solve. another reason for controlling abnormal production of insulin is that it is an inflammatory which is directly linked to cancer as well as arterial inflammation which allows cholesterol to adhere to the inside of the arteries, the cure for this one is usually very easy. Just stop consuming any kind of sugar or high glycemic index carbohydrates and starches. You will find more on this subject at the end of the book.

If you need to take calcium channel blockers it indicates that you have insufficient magnesium in your system because magnesium is what keeps the calcium from entering the cell in the first place. Whenever calcium is needed within a cell the magnesium molecule knows to get out of the way and allow the calcium to enter. When enough calcium has entered the cell the magnesium resumes its duty of restricting its intake. so before you go on a calcium channel blocker try at least 500 mg of magnesium gluconate per day and see if that doesn't cure the problem. You should keep in mind that magnesium is a laxative so if you consume more than 500 mg per day it may be a problem. Fortunately there are several companies who produce a topical version of magnesium, which you can moisten and rub onto your skin and it will be absorbed directly into your bloodstream. Another way of accomplishing the same thing  is to place a crushed up magnesium tablet between your lower lip and gum like it was snuff. This will allow it to be absorbed directly into your bloodstream and bypass your digestive system.

## Mandatory Supplementation

The medications that where prescribed to you by your cardiologist will keep your symptoms under control. If however you want a substantial increase in ejection fraction you will need to take the following supplements. They are what cured me in 6 months. An ailing heart is much less efficient than a healthy one at absorbing nutrients from the blood plasma. For that reason we need to make it as easy as possible for sick heart muscle cells to easily acquire the nutrients that they needs by consuming relatively high daily doses.

**Multi-Vitamin:** One per day

**Vitamin C:** 1,000mg per day

Double blind studies indicate that 1g per day for 4-6 months significantly reduced blood pressure. Lancet 1999;11:405-412 hypertension 2002;40:804-809

**Berberine:** Have not used this plant based supplement so do not know what dosage to recommend. It does seem to have a very good reputation for safety and efficacy when treating high blood pressure.

**CoQ10:** 600mg per day

Double blind studies indicate that 150mg day decreased BP by 18/12 after 1-4 months. Also improves cell mitochondrial and heart function. Southern medical journal 2001;1112-1117

**D-Ribose:** 15g per day

There are no natural sources for this so your body must

synthesize it and there is never enough. It is used by our DNA RNA as well as ATP, which every muscle of our bodies uses to produce energy.

**Vitamin E:** 400iu per day

Do not take the usual form of vitamin E that only contains Alpha-Tocopherol. The other three isomers of natural vitamin E are the Beta, Gama and Delta types of Tocopherol. Gama-Tocopherol is very heart protective but when the Alpha version is ingested by itself it bonds with the Gama-Tocopherol that is already present in our bodies so that there is no free Gama-Tocopherol to help our hearts. Only use vitamin E supplements that contain all four types.

In a recent double blind study of people with risk factors for heart disease who took 400iu of Alpha-Tocopherol vitamin E per day for seven years. There was a 40% increase in the number of hospitalizations and a 19% increase in heart failures over the control group. Not a very good advertisement for taking the Alpha-Tocopherol version of vitamin E! Also be aware that vitamin E and fish oil are also blood thinners, which can cause excessive thinning when used in conjunction with prescription blood thinners. This may allow you to reduce the amount of prescription blood thinner that you need to take.

**L-arginine:** 3,000mg per day Peanuts are 33% arginine by weight.

It causes vasodilation, improves cardiac output and Increases endurance and strength. Promotes repair of damaged muscle tissue.

**L-carnitine:** 1,000mg per day

Improves ejection fraction, exercise tolerance and prolongs survival as well as improving fat lose. It also aids in the transport of fatty acids into cells. American Heart journal 2000;139:S120-S123

**Magnesium Gluconate:** 1,000mg per day

CHF patients need at least 1,000mg of magnesium per day. A damaged heart can only absorb 33% as much serum magnesium into the heart muscle as a healthy one. Use the Gluconate version of Magnesium capsules as the heart more readily utilizes it. Research studies have shown that two grams of IV magnesium administered weekly for six weeks produced marked improvement in 80% of CHF patients. Most patients maintained the improvement for at least a year. Thousands of bodily functions depend on magnesium.

**Omega-3 fatty acids:** 2,000mg per day

Fish oil has modest blood pressure lowering effects. Sunflower and safflower oil have a moderate effect. Circulation 1993;88:523-533

**Potassium:** 2,000mg per day

High potassium intake lowers BP and protects against hypertensive effects of salt. Suppresses renin release, increases ureases, relaxes vascular smooth muscle. 3-4 g per day significantly lowers BP. US diet has 1.5 g. Contraindicated in end stage renal disease and patients taking potassium-sparing diuretics

**Resveratrol:** 200mg per day 3x per day between lower lip and gum

This is the only inexpensive easily obtainable supplement that has been proven to lengthen the telomeres on the ends of our DNA thereby lengthening both the quantity and quality of our lives. Recent studies have shown that most of a dose of resveratrol when swallowed is destroyed by the digestive tract. The proper way to take it is to open the capsule and pour the contents into the space between the lower lip and gums where it will be absorbed directly into your blood stream within about 15 minutes. You can then swallow the rest. This will result in a blood level of resveratrol more than 100 times greater than that provided by swallowing a 1,000 mg capsule.

**Selenium:** 300mcg per day (a couple of Brazil nuts will provide it)

**Taurine:** 1,000mg per day

Actively transported into the heart muscle cells at hundreds of times the concentration found in blood plasma. This is a very difficult process for healthy heart cells let alone damaged ones who are usually 60% less efficient at osmosis. This probably means that the heart considers it to be vital for its health. It stabilizes cell membranes in the heart and has inotropic and antiarrhythmic effects. The good news is that four eggs a day will supply the 1,000 mgs.

**Thiamine and B6:** Take a good B complex supplement 150 mg per day

Thiamine deficiency can cause CHF so supplementation is essential. It will increase the need for magnesium so be sure to supplement that as well.

# Foods that have the highest concentrations of nutrients

| | | |
|---|---|---|
| Vitamin A | 1 Sweet Potato | 550% of your DV |
| Vitamin B6 | 1 cup Chickpeas | 55% of your DV |
| Vitamin B12 | one Clam | 1,400% of your DV |
| Vitamin C | one Bell Pepper | 10% of your DV |
| Vitamin D | 1 oz. Cod Liver Oil | 140% of your DV |
| Vitamin E | one oz. Almonds | 37% of your DV |
| Vitamin K | one cup Spinach | 1,000% of your DV |
| Calcium | one cup plain Yogurt | 42% of your DV |
| Folate | one cup Spinach | 65% of your DV |
| Lycopene | one Tomato | 300% of your DV |
| Lysine | two Eggs | 100% of your DV |
| Magnesium | one cup Spinach | 550% of your DV |
| Niacin | one cup Peanuts | 100% of your DV |
| Potassium | one Sweet Potato | 100% of your DV |
| Riboflavin | 3 oz. Liver | 100% of your DV |
| Selenium | one Brazil nut | 100% of your DV |
| Taurine | 4 Eggs | 100% of your DV |
| Zinc | 3 oz. Beef | 100% of your DV |

## Lifestyle Changes

You need to keep an eye on your kidney and liver function. Quite often CHF or the factors that lead up to it will tend to overload them as well causing impaired function. When you get home from the hospital you will also need to be very proactive and figure it all out for yourself. Your cardiologist can prescribe medications to alleviate your symptoms, but will not be able to force you to make the necessary dietary and lifestyle changes that are needed in order to live past that first critical year when 40% of CHF victims die. This Usually occurs because they refuse to stop eating improperly and implement a sensible exercise program to improve their physical conditioning. Your life depends on your ability to reduce unnecessary heart loads such as excess fat tissue and emotional stress.

## Behaviors to eliminate

## Sodium Consumption

You must limit your intake of sodium to 2.5 grams or less per day in order to lower water retention, which increases your blood pressure and edema. This will probably require you to make many of your own cooking ingredients such as tomato paste and mayonnaise from scratch as the commercial ready to use versions have enormous amounts of salt in them. The following types of products contain large amounts of sodium as well.

Processed meat such as sausages and salami.

Many cheeses have high sodium content.

Nuts, Buy the unsalted varieties.

Steak Sauces such as Worcestershire Sauce.

Bouillon Cubes, Soy Sauce and Teriyaki Sauce.

Salad Dressings.

Snack Foods such as potato chips.

Even if there is a label on the front of a package that says reduced sodium, check the ingredients label to see what the reality is. Watch out for different forms of sodium such as sodium citrate, which is just as dangerous as sodium chloride (table salt). If the word sodium is listed on the ingredients label, in whatever form, you need to determine exactly how much that product contains. Become obsessed with reading ingredients labels on processed food packages. You will be amazed at the amount of salt contained in many of them.

1/4 teaspoon salt = 575 mg sodium

1/2 teaspoon salt = 1,150 mg sodium

3/4 teaspoon salt = 1,725 mg sodium

1 teaspoon salt  = 2,300 mg sodium

Mrs. Dash produces a very good seasoning that is salt free. You can find it in the spice section of your food market or on Amazon.com.

## Fast Food

Fast food has a very high level of salt and unhealthy fats not to mention being made from the lowest quality ingredients available. Try the Mediterranean diet. You can prepare it yourself and save a lot of money. Studies have shown it to reduce the chance of recurring heart attack mortality by as much as 70%.

## Smoking

Smoking reduces the amount of oxygen in the blood increasing the workload on your heart. It also constricts your blood vessels.

## Alcohol

If your CHF is not sever an occasional glass of wine or a small beer probably will not be a problem. If you do not have sufficient will power to limit your intake then don't start! This can be a problem for me down here in South America where we have some of the world's best wine.

## All Sugars

Stop eating sugar in any form or quantity and substitute powdered stevia instead. It has zero calories and tastes like real sugar. The ones from Bolivia are the best with no bitter after taste. You only need a very small amount so go easy until you learn how much is needed. The main reason to stop consuming sugar is that it is the worst systemic inflammatory that we eat and is the main cause of both cancer and vascular disease. This inflammation is like taking sandpaper to the inside of your arteries, it or any other inflammatory is what actually causes cholesterol to adhere to the walls of the blood vessels. After your body has gotten over the sugar withdrawal symptoms start eliminating any high glycemic carbohydrates such as milk, white bread and white vegetables.

## Eating at Restaurants

Their job is to sell food not to protect your health. Making the food taste good is their main concern not your health. You can easily consume 3,000mg of sodium in one meal and if you think the waitress will be able to advise you about which menu items are low sodium you had better think again. Even commercial salad dressings have very high concentrations of sodium.

**Green vegetables**

Most of them contain vitamin K which thickens the blood. If you are trying to thin your blood to reduce the load on your heart they should be avoided. Below is a list of low vitamin K foods for people on blood thinners. Being consistent with both the amount of vitamin K consumed and the dosage of blood thinner taken per day is the important part. Warfarin was originally used as a rat poison so limiting your intake would seem to be a good idea as well if possible.

**Vitamin K foods to limit to 1 serving per day (200%-660% DV)**

| Food | Serving | Vitamin K |
|------|---------|-----------|
| Kale | 1/2 cup | (660% DV) |
| Spinach | 1/2 cup | (560% DV) |
| Turnip Greens | 1/2 cup | (530% DV) |
| Collard Greens | 1/2 cup | (520% DV) |
| Swiss Chard | 1/2 cup | (360% DV) |
| Parsley | 1/4 cup | (300% DV) |
| Mustard Greens | 1/2 cup | (260% DV) |

## Vitamin K foods to limit to 3 serving per day (60%-200% DV)

| Food | Serving | Vitamin K |
|---|---|---|
| Brussels Sprouts | 1/2 cup | (190% DV) |
| Spinach | 1 cup | (180% DV) |
| Turnip Greens | 1 cup | (170% DV) |
| Leaf Lettuce | 1 cup | (125% DV) |
| Broccoli | 1 cup | (110% DV) |
| Endive | 1 cup | (70% DV) |
| Romaine Lettuce | 1 cup | (70% DV) |

## Foods Low in Vitamin K to eat when taking Warfarin

| Food | Serving | Vitamin K |
|---|---|---|
| Turnips | 1 cup | 0μg (0% DV) |
| Beets | 1 cup | 0μg (0% DV) |
| Sweet Corn | 1 cup | 0μg (1% DV) |
| Onions | 1 | 1μg (1% DV) |
| Rutabagas | 1 cup | 0μg (1% DV) |
| Pumpkin | 1 cup | 2μg (2% DV) |
| Squash | 1 cup | 2μg (2% DV) |

# Foods Low in Vitamin K to eat when taking Warfarin

| Potatoes | 1 cup | 3μg (4% DV) |
|---|---|---|
| Sweet Potatoes | 1 cup | 7μg (9% DV) |
| Eggplants | 1 cup | 3μg (4% DV) |
| Bamboo shoots | 1 cup | 0μg (0% DV) |
| Mushrooms | 1 cup | 0μg (0% DV) |
| Tomatoes | 1 cup | 7μg (8% DV) |
| Cucumbers | 1 cup | 17μg (21% DV) |
| Iceberg Lettuce | 1 cup | 17μg (22% DV) |
| Artichokes | 1 | 17μg (22% DV) |

# Fruits Low in Vitamin K

| Food | Serving | Vitamin K |
|------|---------|-----------|
| Oranges | 1 | 0µg (0% DV) |
| Watermelon | 1 cup | 0µg (0% DV) |
| Litchis | 1 cup | 0µg (1% DV) |
| Bananas | 1 | 0µg (1% DV) |
| Pineapple | 1 cup | 1µg (1% DV) |
| Apples | 1 | 4µg (5% DV) |
| Nectarines | 1 | 3µg (4% DV) |
| Strawberries | 1 cup | 3µg (4% DV) |
| Peaches | 1 | 4µg (5% DV) |

Avoid grapefruit and cranberries

**All grains are low in vitamin K**

| Food | Serving Size | Vitamin K |
|------|--------------|-----------|
| White Rice | 1 cup | 0μg (0% DV) |
| Brown Rice | 1 cup | 1.2μg (1% DV) |
| Couscous | 1 cup | 0.2μg (0% DV) |
| Cornmeal | 1 cup | 0.4μg (0% DV) |
| Pearled Barley | 1 cup | 1.3μg (2% DV) |
| Pasta (Plain) | 1 cup | 0μg (0% DV) |
| Whole Wheat Bread | 1 Slice | 0μg (0% DV) |
| Buckwheat | 1 cup | 3.2μg (4% DV) |
| Quinoa | 1 cup | 0.0μg (0% DV) |

**Behaviors to implement**

**Reduce Body Fat**

This is one of the most important lifestyle changes to initiate. Our fat cells are supported by a vast system of capillaries, which impose a substantial load on the heart. If you are truly obese and reduce your body weight by 50% your heart would have 50% less workload, which could very well eliminate most of the symptoms of your CHF.

## Be happy and enjoy life

Depression and stress will kill you faster than anything else. If you have all of your appendages and are able to function normally you have an obligation to everyone around you to be happy and an inspiration to those who are less able to cope with their physical or emotional problems.

## Learn to cook

Preparing your own food is the best way to insure that it has no harmful ingredients. The meals you prepare will also be richer in vitamins and minerals. If you need a chemistry degree to read the ingredients label on a product then don't buy it. I am really enjoying making my own meals from scratch and having complete control over the kinds of food that go into my body. Intelligent food preparation is a very enjoyable way to spend some of your free time and it will go a long way towards eliminating CHF symptoms. It is much more economical as well.

## Exercise

As I have previously stated our physiological characteristics were set a million or so years in the past when our survival depended mainly upon our ability to find food and to escape from predators. Evolutionary success always seems to be a balance between too little and too much of a good thing. Too little food and we died of starvation, too much caused us to become over weight and we couldn't run and climb fast enough to escape from predators. Too much muscle caused a similar problem, we became stronger but also heavier and were no longer able to climb or run fast enough to escape from those same predators.

So far as evolution was concerned as long as we managed to have children and raise them we had fulfilled our evolutionary purpose and became expendable. This usually occurred at around 30 years of age at most so evolution never had a reason to extend our lives any further. If the genes we passed on to our progeny had positive survival characteristics they in turn would survive longer, have more progeny and pass those same positive genes on to their offspring. And so it continued for millennia until our physiologies had been refined to the point where our bodies were completely adapted to survival in the existing environment. So long as the environment did not change we were in perfect harmony with it and our physical health was assured. Unfortunately since the beginning of the 19th century technological evolution has progressed much faster than our biological evolutionary process could keep up with.

The second factor that regulated muscle growth was that muscle requires the expenditure of large amounts of energy to maintain. This is the reason our bodies do not want us to acquire more muscle than we absolutely need to survive and why it is so difficult to acquire muscle through exercise. There is no one exercise program that will suit all CHF patients. I am an extreme example to use but it may give you some idea of what a bodybuilder with CHF is capable of. I have been lifting weights consistently for the last 40 years. I am 66 years old 5' 8" tall and weigh 175 lbs with 12% body fat, which I am currently reducing down to 8% to remove as much load from my heart as possible. Because of the growing amount of obesity in western society CHF has become an ever more popular area of research. Many of these studies have been done comparing the relative benefits of cardio verses weight lifting for recovering CHF patients. Most indicate that weight training is superior to cardio in this regard because it preserves muscle mass as well as providing aerobic conditioning.

Walking is great exercise as well. You can vary the resistance by how fast you walk and how steep the grade is that you are walking up. You can also pick a different location each time to vary the scenery. I would not limit myself to the inside of a mall on the assumption that if you had a heart attack that someone would save you. The odds of someone around you having been trained in CPR are very small and only 5% of CPR recipients survive longer than half an hour. If you have an ICD implanted it will get your heart going again much more efficiently than any paramedic and much quicker.

I walk a mile to the local gym here in Arequipa every other day to lift weights. The only difference between now and before my heart attack is that I need to rest for two minutes between exercise sets to catch my breath instead of only one. I do about an hour of maximum effort lifting, usually combination exercises that work muscle groups prior to walking the mile back to my apartment. Weight training if done properly is just as aerobic as running. If not then you are not using enough weight or repetitions or are resting too long between sets.

## Could Have, Should Have, Would have

The early stages of my CHF probably were present three or more years ago when I first came to Arequipa, Peru. Although I didn't develop any obvious symptoms of altitude sickness, I noticed that I did not develop increased endurance after a month of acclimation. Also I have had very low levels of edema around my ankles for years. This I believe was due to chronic high blood pressure as well as lack of proper nutrition for an extended period of time causing my systemic levels of D-Ribose to drop.

I have always had a problem with fat. As a result of this I tended to stay on a high protein low carbohydrate diet for extended periods of time, relying on protein shakes and vitamins. This probably deprived my body of the nutrients it needed to manufacture sufficient amounts of D-Ribose allowing my body's level to become insufficient to maintain heart health. Eventually when my heart attack occurred my heart muscle cells were unable to recover and remained in a state of hibernation even after the coronary blockage was removed and normal blood flow was restored to them. When they finally started receiving enough of the nutrients they needed most of them came back on line and started functioning again.

The side effects of ACE inhibitors are almost nonexistent so if your blood pressure has started going up, taking a small dose every day might be a way of preventing cumulative damage over time. My blood pressure was 140/85 for a number of years and I have to wonder how much of a factor it was in my CHF. Not only is your heart health at risk but also the health of your liver and kidneys as well. That is a Trifecta that you cannot afford to loose! These are the three most important organs in your body and high blood pressure damages all of them. Judging by my own Bun and Creatinine numbers I will probably die of liver or kidney failure before my heart gets its chance to do me in. So being proactive and a little too early with blood pressure intervention is probably the best course to take. I certainly wish I had.


## My Routine

Sufficient sleep is vital for your health even under the best of circumstances, and I can assure you that suffering from CHF does not qualify you for the best of circumstances category. If you are having trouble getting to sleep make sure that there is no light entering your bedroom. Our bodies still operate the same way they did a million years ago and there was no electric lighting or computer monitors back then to interrupt our natural sleep patterns. If our brains sense any light they assume that it is sunrise and release serotonin, which stimulates us to become active. Melatonin is released when it is dark to promote sleep. Older people may have low melatonin levels and need supplementation of 1-3mg. Go to bed early. One hour of sleep before midnight is worth two hours after midnight.

I usually get up about 5:00 am, walk to the gym at 6:00 and lift weights until 7:30 then walk back to my apartment. I also have kettle bells and a high bar at the apartment for days that I can't make it to the gym. Last year my body stopped production of Testosterone so I need to inject 25mg per day. I also inject 100mcg each of Mod GRF (1-29) and GHRP-2 to stimulate the release of about 4iu of growth hormone from my pituitary each day.

The end result is that I have twice as much of these two vital hormones as a 20 year old. I have been supplementing my natural production of Growth Hormone for the last ten years. During the four months that I was having cosmetic surgery performed I had been injecting the peptides twice per day to reduce scarring. I mention all of this because it may have been a factor in both the speed and quality of my recovery. This is one of the reasons that I live in South America where all medications are over the counter and do not require a prescription. One benefit of high levels of Testosterone is that it increases oxygen utilization as well as muscle efficiency. This helps compensate for the high altitude I am currently living at. And would probably increase respiratory efficiency at sea level as well.

Exercise seems to have the most positive effect on edema. On days that I go to the gym I have 70% less edema in my lower calves throughout the day. This effect lasts for the remainder of the day even when sitting at a computer terminal for 12 hours and receiving no further exercise. For some reason I have no arterial stenosis even though I am 66 years old. This of course allows my heart to function more efficiently than would otherwise be the case. Unfortunately without performing very expensive testing I cannot provide any quantitative information about physical improvements in my heart structure that might be contributing to my steady improvement.

Much of my success is probably due to equal parts of luck, genetics and being in good physical condition when the heart attack occurred.

## Fat Loss strategies

Under the best of circumstances there is a 40% chance you will die within the next year so don't push your luck! If you don't want to become a Darwin Award nominee the first thing you need to do is decide not to be a part of that statistic. The second thing is to stop eating sugar in any form or quantity, substitute powdered stevia instead. It is not necessary to give up eating sweet food it is only necessary to stop using sugar to produce that sweetness. The main reason for doing this has nothing to do with your being fat or not. The main reason to stop consuming sugar is that it's the worst systemic inflammatory that we consume and is one of the primary causes of both cancer and vascular disease. This inflammation is like taking sandpaper to the inside of your arteries, it or any other inflammatory is what actually causes cholesterol to adhere to the walls of the blood vessels. Loose the sugar and you will loose a significant amount of arterial plaque.

A couple of years ago when I was shopping in Costco I noticed a display of diet drink. Out of curiosity I picked up one of the cans and read the labeling. Prominently displayed on the front of the can in a couple of different locations were the words "Contains zero fat!" When I turned the can over and read the ingredients label I found that it did indeed contain no fat because the main ingredient was sugar! The terrifying thing about this is that there are literally millions of nutritionally ignorant people out there who actually believe that eating fat will make you fat and consuming sugar will not.

## Ketogenesis and Fat loss

Our bodies were designed for life, as it was 100,000 or more years ago. Agriculture had not been invented yet so there was no continuous supply of calories available to keep us going. We were hunter-gatherers who might have a surplus of food one day and none for the next four. To cope with this our bodies developed the ability to store energy in the form of fat and then utilize that stored energy for fuel when no food was available.

Carbohydrates in whatever form are first used to make blood glucose. When our bodies have enough to supply our current energy needs, the remainder is turned into fat for future use. There are only two types of sugar that can cross the brain blood barrier and nourish it, Glucose and ketones. After about 14 hours without carbohydrates our blood glucose levels become low enough that our bodies switch over to converting our fat stores to ketones. Obviously blood glucose depletion happened on a regular basis when we were hunter-gatherers. This was not normally a problem since our bodies would simply switch over to converting fat to ketones, which then were used by our bodies for energy until such time as we were able to find a source of food and once again increase our blood glucose to high levels, and if we were lucky we would have enough left over to store some as fat for later use.

A good analogy is an automobile's gas tank. When we fill it up we are limited to the capacity of the tank. Normally we do not keep trying to put gas in if it keeps running back out the filler pipe onto the ground. We then drive the car using the gasoline stored in it's tank until such time as the tank is close to empty when we fill it again and repeat the cycle. It is the same with our bodies, our fat cells are our gas tank and we convert the fat in them to ketones as we look for more food to replenish our fat stores so that they can provide energy in the future when we can't locate a source of food. Unfortunately our bodies have a limitless gas tank. They simply add more fat cells to contain any extra carbohydrates that we consume. Our fat cells are the perennial pessimists of our bodies and are always preparing for the next famine.

Until recently our systemic levels of glucose have always been very low. Because carbohydrates and pure sugars were so difficult to find our diets consisted mainly of proteins and fats, which supplied our immediate energy needs but could not be stored for future use. Sugars were in the form of fruit, which was often out of season and honey, which was very dangerous to collect. To compensate for this our bodies developed an insatiable craving for anything sweet because it could be easily converted directly into fat so that we would have reserves of energy to fall back on during the lean times.

Fast forward to the modern era. We use fewer calories to maintain our bodies because of our easier workloads but at the same time we have readily available sources of cheap high glycemic food to store as fat. This makes our bodies very happy because they have an endless supply of carbohydrates to convert into fat for the future famine, which never comes. We have so lost touch with reality that we think that being in ketosis is a bad thing that can be solved by simply eating something. In reality having low blood glucose and using our fat stores for energy is historically our normal state and not something to be avoided.

Ketogenic diets are very effective for fat lose and many of the recipes are delicious as well as easy to make. Because of the richness and caloric density of Ketogenic foods you will eat less often and consume a much smaller quantity at each meal. When we are in ketosis 50-70% of our calories should come from good fats such as the medium chain triglycerides found in coconut oil and avocados. This high concentration of beneficial fats and proteins instead of high glycemic carbohydrates makes it easier for our bodies to switch over to burning our stored fat when the food in our stomach has been consumed. I view the hard core Ketogenic diet as a temporary diet to loose large quantities of fat quickly, after which you can switch to a more varied one such as the Mediterranean diet, which has been proven to reduce death in heart attack victims by 70%.


## Mediterranean Diet

The Mediterranean diet is currently one of the most popular and with good reason. Greek and Turkish foods are amongst the most flavorful in the world. This is a great maintenance diet once you have lost your fat. Just don't use it as an excuse to pig out on pasta and regain the fat that you have lost. Some of the benefits are:

1. Provides quick weight loss.

2. There are many high protein and fat dishes.

3. A small amount is very filling.

4. It helps maintain low blood sugar levels.

5. It is simple to prepare.

6. People with elevated levels of insulin tend to see reductions.

There is even a Ketogenic version that can be found here: www.advancedmediteranean.com


## Intermittent Fasting

Intermittent fasting is a great tool for loosing fat and is very synergistic when combined with the Ketogenic diet. You eat dinner a couple of hours before going to bed. If you eat at 7:00 pm and go to bed at 10:00 pm for example you would wake at around 6:00 am. At this point you have been fasting for 11 hours and your goal is to not consume anything but water until around 2:00 am in the afternoon.

At this point you will have fasted for 19 hours and you can then eat enough Ketogenic food to just satisfy your immediate hunger so that you can make it to 7:00 pm for your next Ketogenic dinner just prior to bedtime. Combining a Ketogenic diet with intermittent fasting is one of the quickest and most effective means of loosing fat, especially if you are getting regular exercise as well. The website www.leangains.com is the place to go for information on this type of fat loss.


## Fat Cell Apoptosis

If you follow the advice about ketogenic dieting and intermittent fasting you will probably find that you initially lose a very large volume of fat but that when you have lost about two thirds of the fat you started out with you suddenly stopped losing the remaining 30%. There is a very simple and logical reason for this. At this point you have very little fat stored in the remaining fat cells. They are empty but like empty one liter water bottles the cells still take up space. It is only possible to lose two thirds of your fat volume by dieting alone.

At this point you need to wait until your body decides that you no longer will need those empty fat cells for future fat storage. The problem is that our bodies are programed to expend as little energy as possible and preemptively destroying all of those billions of fat cells would require the expenditure of a great deal of energy. The end result is that our bodies take a wait and see approach and allow the fat cells to die of old age rather than taking an active role in eliminating them. Since all of the cells in our bodies are replaced approximately every 3 to 5 years that much time will have to pass before all of those unused fat cells are eliminated.

This does not mean that you will carry the remaining empty fat cells for five years at which point they will all disappear overnight. Some have already reached the end of their useful life span and will immediately begin to die. so it will probably take you three years to lose most of the remaining bulge around your waist. A big problem with trying to lose fat around your waist is that our bodies want to keep it not just as a source of energy but also to protect our vital internal organs from cold weather. Fat is an excellent insulation so our bodies first eliminate all fat from our appendages arms, legs and face before using the fat that is stored around our torsos. All of this can be very frustrating and cause the person to give up and go back to eating the same as they did prior to losing the fat which of course causes them to gain all of the fat back again. This is why any form of diet change has to involve lifestyle and mental changes as well. It has to go all the way to the core of your being and not just be a superficial attempt at improving your figure. It is a fact that all healthy diets no matter of what type will produce dramatic fat loss. What people have to understand is that it is not a steady-state and that your strategy needs to change along with your current metabolic situation. My advice to people who want to improve their physiques is that they will gain more muscle and loose more fat by reading about the process than actually going to a gym and working out. What I mean of course is that you have to be smarter than your body on this subject, and your body has a million year head start on you!

## Ketogenic Recipes

Here are some standard Keto recipes to get you started. They are mostly desserts and all of them taste like their high carb relatives but eating them will cause you to loose fat.

## Avocado Mint Chocolate Chunk Ice Cream

I make 4 kilos at a time and freeze it in small containers.

### Ingredients

Mint flavoring to taste (preferably natural white powdered mint)

Vanilla flavoring to taste (preferably natural white powdered vanilla)

2 ripe avocados

1-cup coconut milk

Half-cup heavy cream

Half-cup of unsweetened baker's chocolate cut into 1/4" chunks. (approximate size)

Sweeten to taste with powdered stevia

### Preparation

1. Cut the avocados in half and scoop their insides into a bowl.

2. Add the cup of coconut milk, half cup of heavy cream and 2 tsp. Vanilla.

3. Blend this mixture together until smooth and creamy.

4. Blend the chocolate chunks and stevia into the avocado mixture.

5. Put the bowl in the freezer for about 10 hours to freeze.

6. Remove from Freezer 40 minutes prior to eating so that it can soften.


## Keto Maple Syrup

### Ingredients

3/4 Cup of water

1 Tbsp. of unsalted butter

2 1/4 tsp. Coconut Oil

2 tsp. maple extract

1/2 tsp. vanilla Extract

1/4 tsp. xanthan gum to thicken

Sweeten to taste with stevia

### Preparation

1. Mix your butter, coconut oil, and xanthan gum together in a microwave safe container.

2. Microwave the mixture for 40-50 seconds.

3. Mix microwaved oils and water together.

4. Add vanilla and maple extract and powdered stevia to taste. Thin with water if needed.

5. Microwave for 40-60 seconds, stir, and let cool.

## Keto Pancakes

### Ingredients

4 Tbsp. Heavy Cream

4 Tbsps. of flax seed

2 Eggs

2 Tbsps. Peanut Butter

2 Tbsps. Keto Maple Syrup

1/2 tsp. baking powder

1 Tbsp. Butter

### Preparation

1. Mix Peanut Butter, Maple Syrup, and eggs together.

2. Add the 4 Tbsp. Heavy Cream.

3. Mix in the flax seed and baking powder.

4. Grease a pan with butter at medium heat.

5. Cook the pancakes until the tops bubble then flip over. Cook for an additional 1-2 minutes.


## Strawberry Preserves

### Ingredients

16 oz. Fresh Strawberries

Powdered Stevia

5 tbsp. Chia Seeds

**Preparation**

1. Slice the strawberries into small pieces.

2. Place strawberries in a pan over medium heat.

3. Let it boil for about 5 minutes, until the juice has thickened slightly.

4. Add the chia seeds and stir for about 2 minutes. Remove from heat and let cool. The Chia Seeds produce a coating of gel when in contact with liquid. They will thicken the jam and are very good for you as well.


**Strawberry Milk Shake**

**Ingredients**

1 cup Coconut Milk

1/2 cup Heavy Cream

1/4 cup Milk

4 tbsps. of the keto strawberry jam

2 tbsps. coconut oil

4 Ice Cubes

**Preparation**

Place the ingredients in a blender. Blend to the consistency you want. The strawberries will cause the milk to thicken so if you want a thicker shake add more strawberries and milk.

# Keto Chocolate Chip Cookies (2g Net carbs per cookie)

## Ingredients

1-1/2 cups Almond Flour

5 tbsp. powdered egg whites

3 tbsp. Coconut Flour

3 tbsp. Psyllium Husk

10 tbsp. Unsalted Butter

3 tsp. Vanilla Extract

1 tsp. Baking Powder

2 Eggs

1 bar Unsweetened Chocolate diced into small pieces.

Powdered Stevia.

## Preparation

1. Mix dry ingredients together.

2. Beat warm butter with an electric mixer for 2 minutes.

3. Add the egg and vanilla to the butter and beat until combined.

4. Sift the dry ingredients over the wet ones and mix well.

5. Mix the chocolate chips into dough. Divide the dough into 22 equal pieces.

6. Roll dough into balls, place on a cookie sheet and flatten.

7. Preheat oven to 350F and Bake for 15 minutes.

**Ketogenic BBQ pulled chicken breast**

**Ingredients**

2 boneless skinless chicken breasts.

3 cups tomato sauce

6 finely chopped garlic cloves

1 finely chopped onion

9 tablespoons cider vinegar

3 tablespoons Worcestershire sauce

3 teaspoons paprika

2 teaspoons freshly ground black pepper

2 teaspoons chili powder

1 teaspoon celery seeds

Add Stevia to taste

**Preparation**

1. Mix ingredients, except chicken, in a small pot over medium heat until they come to a boil.

2. Add Stevia and vinegar for sweet sour taste.

3. Add the boneless skinless chicken breasts and let simmer about an hour until very tender.

4. Use a couple of forks to shred the chicken breasts.

## Thai Sweet and Sour Cucumber and Onion Salad

### Ingredients

4 Large Cucumbers, unpeeled and sliced

2 Red Onions, sliced

2 Cup White Vinegar

1 Cup water

Sweeten to taste with Powdered Stevia

### Preparation

1. Prepare the cucumbers and onions. Place them in a Tupperware container that has a secure lid.

2. Add the other ingredients.

3. Add more vinegar to increase the sour flavor, more Stevia to increase the sweetness or water to reduce both. Let it marinate for a few hours in the refrigerator and serve. If you let it marinate long enough the cucumber slices turn into pickles. I then add dill and clove to make dill pickles.

# A Short History of Heart Failure Treatment

## Early Greeks 5th-3rd Century BC

The clinical texts attributed to Hippocrates, describe patients with shortness of breath and edema. However many of these patients probably suffered from conditions other than heart failure. Without a basic knowledge of circulatory function they were unable to attribute cause to any observable symptoms. Palpitation and shortness of breath were attributed to the passage of phlegm, from the brain into the chest.

## Alexandria, Egypt 3rd Century BC

Herophilus and Erasistratus understood that the heart contracts, as well as the function of the valves, they still did not understand that the heart is a pump that circulates the blood.

## Roman Empire 2nd Century BC

Galen, a Greek physician who lived in the Roman Empire during the second century knew that the volume of the heart decreases during heart contraction and understood the function of the heart's valves, but viewed the heart as a heat source rather than a pump. This basic lack of knowledge about the true function of the heart of course made it impossible to understand the causes and symptoms of heart malfunction let alone provide treatments. This lack of knowledge caused heart failure symptoms to be treated with the following remedy.

"Take scabwort and grind and squeeze its juice through a cloth, collect in an eggshell and temper with honeycomb; give the patient daily a full shell of the juice, do this for eleven days when the moon is waning because also man wanes in his abdomen."


## Heart Disease as a Circulatory Disorder 1600s

Physicians started to perform autopsies to identify causes of illness. Because of this, cardiac abnormalities began to be associated with their clinical manifestations when the patients were alive. There still was no way to define the connection between the clinical and autopsy findings in patients with heart failure until 1628 when William Harvey described the circulation of blood through our bodies.

"I am obliged to conclude that in animals the blood is driven round a circuit with an unceasing, circular sort of movement that this is an activity or function of the heart which it carries out by virtue of its pulsation, and that in sum it constitutes the sole reason for that heart's pulsatile movement."


## The Structural Differences of Failed Hearts 1700s

Physicians began to have a better understanding of the structural changes that occur in a failing heart. Lancisi, in 1707, distinguished between "dilation" of a ventricle, where cavity size is increased, and "hypertrophy", where the wall thickness of the ventricle increases but the chamber becomes smaller. In 1759 Morgagni described the link between high blood pressure and hypertrophy of ventricles. The century that followed was focused on structural changes in the failing heart.

## The Study of Blood Pressure Abnormalities 1800s

Hemodynamics remained central for understanding heart failure throughout the first half of the eighteenth century, when most patients with heart disease had structural abnormalities caused by rheumatic fever, syphilis, and congenital disorders.

## Biochemical Treatments 1900s

It wasn't until the early 1940s, when Cardiologists began using cardiac catheterization made it possible to alleviate many forms of structural heart disease. However because of the increased life span of the general population heart attacks and the weakened hearts they produce were on the increase and congestive heart failure became the next problem to solve.

## Controlling Edema 1950s

Since the time of Hippocrates shortness of breath and edema caused suffering that is unknown today. Although physicians as early as the 16th century had suggested excessive fluid as a cause, there had been no safe way to get rid of it until 1920, when some natural diuretics began to be used on CHF patients. Subsequent efforts to develop more powerful diuretics ended successfully in the 1960s with the introduction of the thiazides and loop diuretics. With the virtual elimination of the congestion and edema symptoms researchers were able to focus on increasing the efficiency of the damaged heart itself.

## The Biochemical Era 1960s

During the 1950s biochemical research led to an expansion of understanding in a couple of important areas. Cardiologists who realized that improving the quality of a heart's contraction was the key to improving its function adopted an improved understanding of muscle contraction and relaxation. The second area, was an improved understanding of how enzymes, and hormones bind with receptors and more importantly how to prevent them from doing so lead to the development of beta blockers and ACE inhibitors that are so beneficial for CHF victims today

## Supplemental Deficiencies

One of the most beneficial discoveries was that heart muscles and muscles in general often do not function at full capacity due to an insufficiency of energy producing vitamins, minerals and enzymes. This has lead to efforts focused on optimizing heart muscle strength by making sure that sufficient quantities of these nutrients are present in the blood plasma of CHF patients that their heart muscles are able to obtain enough to fuel function at 100% capacity and have enough left over to repair damaged muscle cells.

## Impairment of Contractility

It has been show that contractility is reduced in patients with chronic heart failure. This is caused both by having fewer functional muscle cells to pump blood through the body but also because of a lack of sufficient nutrients to supply them. An impaired fill rate when the heart relaxes creates as much of a problem as insufficient contractility.

## Stimulation of Neural receptors 1980s

In 1983 the detrimental effects due to the increased activity of the sympathetic nervous system, renin-angiotensin system and vasopressin, which cause vasoconstriction along with salt and water retention was understood. These autonomic responses are one of the main contributors to the transition from ventricular dysfunction to clinical heart failure.

Because vasoconstriction increases cardiac energy expenditure and reduces cardiac output researchers tested long term use of vasodilators. These trials indicated that long term use of dilators can worsen CHF not help it. This suggested that the dramatic benefits of angiotensin II–converting enzyme (ACE) inhibitors were due to factors other than their ability to reduce after-load.

## Hypertrophy 1990s

By the late 1980s, further research revealed some findings indicating that direct-acting vasodilators can worsen prognosis, and a central role for depressed contractility became untenable when inotropes were found to shorten survival. The use of diuretics, vasodilators, and inotropes to treat heart failure was so effective that it was generally believed that the problem of CHF had been solved. Then came the clinical trials that showed that although the short-term prognosis for this treatment regime was very good the long-term survival rate was very poor. An understanding of these apparently counter intuitive findings emerged in the 1990s, when new data from the expanding fields of molecular biology rekindled interest in the deleterious effects of cardiac hypertrophy.

## ABOUT THE AUTHOR

I'm a 66-year-old 5'8" 170lb. bodybuilder. During the last year I have had 4 different facelift procedures done in Thailand, a massive heart attack while under sedation followed by 2.5 hours of CPR and a one-week coma. A month later my weakened heart went into congestive failure so severe that I could not walk 15 feet without being out of breath. Along the way I went through a divorce after being married for 30 years and 3 basal cell carcinomas. I should have died many times over but having decided that there was no viable up side to that strategy I did my research and found cures for all of my afflictions, well...except for the divorce, that one just keeps on giving.

Only 5% of CPR recipients survive longer than 30 minutes. That must put me in the 1% group. Only 50% of extended coma victims survive. 40% of all congestive heart failure patients die within the first year. I currently walk a mile to the gym every other day, lift the same weights as prior to my CHF and then walk back to my apartment. Additionally I walk a couple of more miles each day to shop or visit friends. All of this is in Arequipa, Peru at an altitude of 7,500' where there is 17% less oxygen per breath. I'm a serial survivor who should have died many times over and I have been trying to analyze and quantify the why of it ever since.

Made in the USA
Las Vegas, NV
19 March 2024

87444147R00069